Enhancing Pain Control for Children

BY
Y.DAWSON

CONTENTS Page

ABSTRACT

Over the last 20 years it has been realised that neonates, infants and children experience pain and considerable stress responses to surgical and medical procedures which are harmful and cause fear, anxiety and distress(Walker, 2008).

This thesis will describe a body of work published since 1992 whose aim has been to improve several aspects of pain management for children in terms of both efficacy and safety. The studies encompass research into the four main classes of analgesics used in paediatric clinical practice, namely local anaesthetics, opioids, non-steroidal anti-inflammatory drugs (NSAIDs) and paracetamol. In addition, control of the stress responses to tracheal intubation and to surgery has been studied with the availability of newer potent short-acting opioid agents and the anaesthetic agent propofol. The total body of work described covers 41 peer reviewed publications with 14 index papers selected for more detailed consideration.

Local anaesthetics

Several studies included in this thesis demonstrate the efficacy and safety of local anaesthetics in children.

The optimum dose of the amide local anaesthetic, lignocaine, was determined for preventing pain on intravenous injection of propofol in children(Cameron et al., 1992) and this resulted in the widespread adoption of propofol as an induction agent. Several studies of propofol in children were conducted and this led to the development of more accurate computer-controlled delivery for maintenance of anaesthesia in children down to age 1 year(Morton et al., 1988, Marsh et al., 1990, Morton, 1990a, Marsh et al., 1991, Doyle et al., 1993c, Runcie et al., 1993, Morton, 1998b, Varveris and Morton, 2002).

Topical amethocaine (as a gel and as a phase-change patch) was evaluated in children(Doyle et al., 1993a, Lawson et al., 1995, Lawson and Morton, 1998) and found to have a significantly more rapid onset of action than EMLA cream. This gel is now widely used in the UK.

For nerve block, the efficacy and safety of fascia iliaca compartment block in children was demonstrated(Doyle et al., 1997) and the additional safety margin provided by adding the vasoconstrictor adrenaline to the local anaesthetic solution was proved by very low peak plasma concentrations of local anaesthetic. This was also demonstrated for caudal epidural blockade in infants(Hansen et al., 2001).

New amide local anaesthetics were introduced in the last decade and ropivacaine was shown to be safe and effective for caudal epidural blockade in children(Ivani et al., 1998a). A collaboration with Strathclyde University led to the development of a new micro-assay method for measurement of local anaesthetics in small volumes of plasma with applicability to neonatal age groups of patients where ethically allowable blood sampling volumes are very small(Stumpe et al., 2000).

Opioids

The technique of patient-controlled analgesia was studied in children with an open feasibility trial in 1990(Lawrie et al., 1990) using conventional electronic syringe pumps and a further innovative study of a disposable elastomeric reservoir device in 1992(Irwin et al., 1992). The optimum regimen for PCA in children was determined by a series of studies(Doyle et al., 1994a, Doyle et al., 1993d, Doyle et al., 1994c, Munro et al., 2002) and a subsequent trial demonstrated that PCA could be delivered by the subcutaneous route(Doyle et al., 1994b). A further collaboration with Strathclyde produced a microassay method for morphine and metabolites(Watson et al., 1995). These studies showed that PCA is very efficacious and safe for perioperative pain conrol in children from age 5 years upwards and this technique is now in routine use worldwide(Walker, 2008, APAGBI, 2008, Morton, 2007, Lonnqvist and Morton, 2005b).

NSAIDs and Paracetamol

Following the demonstration of the utility of PCA in children, the technique was used to assess the analgesic efficacy of the NSAID diclofenac and paracetamol in children(Morton and O'Brien, 1999). This showed diclofenac to be particularly efficacious in producing a 40% morphine-sparing effect in children. An innovative study of NSAID eye drops showed them to be as effective as local anaesthetic eye drops for providing analgesia after strabismus surgery in children(Morton et al., 1997).

Dosing regimens for paracetamol have evolved in the last decade based on better information on developmental pharmacokinetics and elucidation of the mechanism of action(Arana et al., 2001, Ottani et al., 2006, Pickering et al., 2006, Anderson and Palmer, 2006). There is renewed interest in this decade with the availability of new IV formulations of this old drug. In 1999(Hansen et al., 1999) we contributed to the PK data for paracetamol in neonates and infants which was subsequently used by authors from New Zealand to determine the population PK parameters in this young age group(Anderson and Palmer, 2006). We collated the knowledge on dosing regimens in 2001 in a review(Arana et al., 2001) which has informed the current recommendations in the BNFC. A further collaboration with Strathclyde University led to the development of a microassay for paracetamol and its metabolites from blood spots which has been taken up by Medecins Sans Frontieres as a possible method to use in the field in developing countries(Oliveira et al., 2002). The morphine-sparing efficacy of paracetamol was shown to be less than that due to diclofenac in the study mentioned above under NSAIDs(Morton and O'Brien, 1999).

Controlling the stress response

Noxious stimuli produce a stress response. A series of studies has shown that using short acting opioids, tracheal intubation could be safely performed without the aid of muscle relaxant drugs in children(Steyn et al., 1994, O'Brien et al., 1998, Robinson et al., 1998). This technique is now widely practiced. Two studies explored methods to reduce the stress response to open heart surgery with cardiopulmonary bypass, one of the most potent surgical stressors. Propofol anaesthesia was shown to significantly ameliorate this response(Laycock et al., 1992) and the newer opioid remifentanil was shown to be as efficacious as the older drug fentanyl for this purpose(Bell et al., 2004).

Audit, guidelines and protocols

Two major analgesic techniques have been audited in large national projects looking at the risk of epidural infusions in children(Llewellyn and Moriarty, 2007) and opioid infusion techniques in children (Morton, 2008c) and the results show these techniques to be of comparable safety. The evidence from the past 20 years has recently been synthesised into a clinical guideline for management of postoperative and procedural pain in children which has highlighted good practice based on high quality evidence but also revealed a paucity of evidence in some fields(APAGBI, 2008). Guidelines for safer paediatric procedural sedation practice is also described(SIGN, 2004, Playfor et al., 2006). The implementation of guidelines relies on the development of a local protocol and the evolution of the acute pain relief service protocol in Glasgow is described.(Morton, 2008a)

- **CHAPTER 1**

Paediatric pain management has developed in the last 20 years in the light of greater understanding of the development of the pain pathways, availability of new drugs and research in paediatric pharmacology. Organisation of the infrastructure to deliver effective pain assessment and pain management has also occurred in the last 15 years with the development of paediatric acute pain teams. These developments are reviewed to place the current thesis in context.

- **CHAPTER 2**

Studies of opioid pharmacokinetics, pharmacodynamics and pharmacogenomics in children are still ongoing and a study of a new micro-assay method for measuring morphine and its metabolites is described(Watson et al., 1995). A new microassay method for measurement of paracaetamol and its metabolites in blood spots is also described which may have utility in neonates and in difficult environments(Oliveira et al., 2002).

- **CHAPTER 3**

Local anaesthesia techniques have wide applicability in paediatrics and are the foundation of the control of procedural, intraoperative and postoperative pain. This chapter describes the first comparative study of amethocaine gel with EMLA cream in children(Lawson et al., 1995), the first study of an innovative phase-change patch formulation of amethocaine in children (Doyle et al., 1993a) and two studies of local anaesthetic pharmacokinetics and dynamics in children(Doyle et al., 1997, Hansen et al., 2001). In addition, the minimal effective dose of lignocaine to abolish injection pain due to propofol is described(Cameron et al., 1992). This allowed more widespread adoption of propofol as an anaesthetic agent in children.

- **CHAPTER 4**

Opioid techniques and regimens suitable for safe use in children have been developed and this chapter describes one index study from a portfolio of studies of patient-controlled analgesia in children(Irwin et al., 1992).

- **CHAPTER 5**

Paracetamol and NSAIDs are commonly used but the evidence base for dosing has until recently been poor, especially in young infants and neonates. A study of paracetamol pharmacokinetics is presented(Hansen et al., 1999) which contributed to more rational dosing regimens in neonates, infants and children. The analgesic efficacy of paracetamol and the NSAID diclofenac was assessed in a study of "morphine-sparing" in children(Morton and O'Brien, 1999).

- **CHAPTER 6**

Stress control for paediatric surgery is particularly important when surgery is major in nature and when patients are young or critically ill. Two studies of control of the stress response to paediatric cardiac surgery are described(Laycock et al., 1992, Bell et al., 2004). Development of techniques of stress free tracheal intubation without the need for muscle relaxants has occurred with the advent of new short-acting opioids. Two studies describe these techniques in children(Steyn et al., 1994, Robinson et al., 1998).

- **CHAPTER 7**

After a large national audit of epidural infusion analgesia in children, the author has led a similar audit of opioid infusion analgesia techniques and the interim results are described in this chapter(Morton, 2008c). The importance of integration and synthesis of the evidence about paediatric analgesia into clinical guidelines and protocols managed by paediatric acute pain teams is emphasised(APAGBI, 2008, Morton, 2008a).

- **CHAPTER 8**

The scientific basis for improving pain control for children is now much more robust and has assumed a much higher priority in care of children undergoing medical and surgical procedures.

INDEX PUBLICATIONS CONSIDERED IN DETAIL

Analgesic assays

Watson DG, Su Q, Midgley JM, Doyle E, Morton NS. Analysis of unconjugated morphine, codeine, normorphine and morphine as glucuronides in small volumes of plasma from children. Journal of Pharmaceutical & Biomedical Analysis. 1995 Jan;13(1):27-32. (Citations 1)

Oliveira EJ, Watson DG, Morton NS. A simple microanalytical technique for the determination of paracetamol and its main metabolites in blood spots. Journal of Pharmaceutical & Biomedical Analysis. 2002 Jul 31;29(5):803-9. (Citations 0)

Local anaesthesia

Cameron E, Johnston G, Crofts S, Morton NS. The minimum effective dose of lignocaine to prevent injection pain due to propofol in children. Anaesthesia. 1992 Jul;47(7):604-6. (Citations 16)

Doyle E, Freeman J, Im NT, Morton NS. An evaluation of a new self-adhesive patch preparation of amethocaine for topical anaesthesia prior to venous cannulation in children. Anaesthesia. 1993 Dec;48(12):1050-2. (Citations 11)

Lawson RA, Smart NG, Gudgeon AC, Morton NS. Evaluation of an amethocaine gel preparation for percutaneous analgesia before venous cannulation in children. British Journal of Anaesthesia. 1995 Sep;75(3):282-5. (Citations 33)

Doyle E, Morton NS, McNicol LR. Plasma bupivacaine levels after fascia iliaca compartment block with and without adrenaline. Paediatric Anaesthesia. 1997;7(2):121-4. (Citations 4)

Hansen TG, Morton NS, Cullen PM, Watson DG. Plasma concentrations and pharmacokinetics of bupivacaine with and without adrenaline following caudal anaesthesia in infants. Acta Anaesthesiologica Scandinavica. 2001 Jan;45(1):42-7. (Citations 6)

Opioids

Irwin M, Gillespie JA, Morton NS. Evaluation of a disposable patient-controlled analgesia device in children.[see comment]. British Journal of Anaesthesia. 1992 Apr;68(4):411-3. (Citations 2)

NSAIDs & paracetamol

Hansen TG, O'Brien K, Morton NS, Rasmussen SN. Plasma paracetamol concentrations and pharmacokinetics following rectal administration in neonates and young infants. Acta Anaesthesiologica Scandinavica. 1999 Sep;43(8):855-9. (Citations 12)

Morton NS, O'Brien K. Analgesic efficacy of paracetamol and diclofenac in children receiving PCA morphine.[see comment]. British Journal of Anaesthesia. 1999 May;82(5):715-7. (Citations 22)

Stress control

Laycock GJ, Mitchell IM, Paton RD, Donaghey SF, Logan RW, Morton NS. EEG burst suppression with propofol during cardiopulmonary bypass in children: a study of the haemodynamic, metabolic and endocrine effects. British Journal of Anaesthesia. 1992 Oct;69(4):356-62. (Citations 2)

Bell G, Dickson U, Arana A, Robinson D, Marshall C, Morton N. Remifentanil vs fentanyl/morphine for pain and stress control during pediatric cardiac surgery. Paediatric Anaesthesia. 2004 Oct;14(10):856-60. (Citations 3)

Steyn MP, Quinn AM, Gillespie JA, Miller DC, Best CJ, Morton NS. Tracheal intubation without neuromuscular block in children.[see comment]. British Journal of Anaesthesia. 1994 Apr;72(4):403-6. (Citations 18)

Robinson DN, O'Brien K, Kumar R, Morton NS. Tracheal intubation without neuromuscular blockade in children: a comparison of propofol combined either with alfentanil or remifentanil. Paediatric Anaesthesia. 1998;8(6):467-71. (Citations 13)

CHAPTER 1:

IMPROVING PAIN MANAGEMENT IN CHILDREN

INTRODUCTION

(APAGBI, 2008, Walker, 2008, Morton, 2007, Harvey and Morton, 2007, SIGN, 2004, Morton, 1998a)

Pain is defined by the International Association for the Study of Pain as *"An unpleasant sensory and emotional experience associated with actual or potential tissue damage or described in terms of such damage"*. There are long-term psychological and physical consequences of inadequate pain control in all age groups (Tables 1.1)(Walker, 2008, Notcutt, 1997).

TABLE 1.1: ADVERSE EFFECTS OF PAIN

PSYCHOLOGICAL	PHYSICAL
anxiety and fear (now and in future)	increased death rate after major surgery
nightmares and sleep disturbance	increased morbidity
behavioural and personality disturbance	*respiratory*: hypoxaemia, impaired respiratory function, decreased cough and cooperation with physiotherapy, increased secretion retention, atelectasis, infection
disruption of schooling	*cardiovascular*: sympathetic stimulation (increased heart rate and blood pressure, vasoconstriction, altered regional blood flow, increased oxygen consumption), risk of venous thrombosis
development of vicious cycles to chronic pain	*stress response*: stress hormone surges, disordered electrolyte and fluid balance, high blood sugar level, osmotic diuresis in neonates, depressed immune function
	cerebral: increase in intracranial pressure, increased risk of intraventicular haemorrhage or cerebral ischaemia in premature neonates
	musculo-skeletal: muscle spasms, immobility, delayed mobilisation
	visceral: slowing of gastrointestinal and urinary function
	wound: decreased healing

LONG-TERM EFFECTS OF PAIN IN EARLY LIFE
alteration in behavioural responses(Grunau et al., 2006)
change in baseline sensory function(Schmelzle-Lubiecki et al., 2007)
enhanced responses to future pain(Taddio et al., 1997, Hermann et al., 2006)
increased analgesic requirements(Peters et al., 2005)

It is now accepted that for moral, humanitarian, ethical and physiological reasons, pain should be anticipated and safely and effectively controlled in all children, whatever their age, maturity or severity of illness (Table 1.2)(Walco et al., 1994).

TABLE 1.2: BENEFITS OF PAIN PREVENTION AND CONTROL

PSYCHOLOGICAL	PHYSICAL
patient satisfaction, reduced anxiety and fear, normalise sleep and behaviour, avoidance of vicious cycles to chronic pain	lower mortality after major surgery, decreased cardiorespiratory complications, earlier weaning from respiratory support, decreased wound and respiratory infection rates, earlier mobilisation and discharge, earlier return of visceral function and oral intake, better fluid and electrolyte homeostasis, reduced cerebral complications

Techniques of pain control should be applied in advance of the painful stimulus wherever possible(RCPCH, 1997, Notcutt, 1997). This pre-emptive approach helps to minimise the emotional problems of fear and anxiety, prevents the "wind-up" phenomenon of central nervous system sensitisation to noxious stimuli and tissue release of pain mediators, ameliorates the stress response, reduces the intraoperative anaesthetic requirement and subsequent analgesic requirements(Walker, 2008, APAGBI, 2008).

A multimodal approach to preventing pain using local anaesthetics, opioids, non-steroidal anti-inflammatory drugs (NSAIDs), sedation and non-drug methods in a safe and effective planned way, tailored to each individual child's needs is the basis of acute pain prevention(Morton, 1998a, Morton, 1993). This requires that pain is assessed regularly and the assessment is linked to action to maintain pain control with minimal adverse effects (APAGBI, 2008, RCN, 1999).

Pain control techniques are not risk-free (Table 1.3)(Llewellyn and Moriarty, 2007, Morton, 2008c)

TABLE 1.3: RISKS OF PAIN CONTROL TECHNIQUES

TECHNIQUE	*INFUSION EQUIPMENT*	*DRUG*
needle damage, misplacement, haematoma, cerebrospinal fluid leak, infection, urinary retention, itch, extravasation of drug, depot effect with subcutaneous/intramuscular route	over-infusion, under-infusion, gravity free-flow, reflux, electronic Interference	allergy, overdose, underdose, prescription error, dilution error, wrong drug, adverse effect

Preparing the child and family in advance with good written and verbal information and careful matching of the analgesic technique to the child will help to reduce fear, anxiety and correct misconceptions. This approach should apply to all painful procedures however minor or major and often means placing pain prevention higher up the list of priorities in each child's overall plan of care. This requires good education of staff, parents and children, forward planning and organisation. A paediatric pain management service has been found to be effective in achieving consistent standards of efficacy and safety (Table 1.4(Lloyd-Thomas and Howard, 1994, Howard, 1996, McKenzie et al., 1997, RCPCH, 1997, Morton, 1998a, Finley and McGrath, 2001, APAGBI, 2008)).

TABLE 1.4: ROLES OF A PAEDIATRIC PAIN MANAGEMENT SERVICE

ORGANISATION	personnel, 24-hour cover, call-out and consultation system, good communication systems, equipment, teaching, clinic for complex/long-term cases
SERVICE DELIVERY	multidisciplinary personnel (pain nurse specialist, anaesthetist, pharmacist, physiotherapist, paediatrician, surgeon, psychologist, psychiatrist, play therapist, etc.), monitoring standard, equipment, follow-up system, daily senior anaesthetic input

EDUCATION	program for anaesthetists, surgeons, paediatricians, emergency room staff, nurses, pharmacists, parents, children, management personnel
AUDIT	efficacy, safety, adverse events, outcome, equipment, costs, efficiency, benefits, risks
RESEARCH	drugs, equipment, monitoring

Studies have shown that one of the major reasons for poor paediatric pain management is a lack of education of staff, parents and children. Myths and misconceptions persist, for example that children do not feel pain as much as adults or are at risk of addiction if opioids are used. Many medical staff are still worried about the safety aspects of prescribing adequate doses of analgesia for children. Medical and nursing students and trainees have often received very little formal training in paediatric pain management but are expected to prescribe and administer analgesia to children. As a result, staff often express undue concern about side effects and tend to use inadequate doses of analgesic drugs. Fears regarding opioid addiction often lead to a change to a weaker analgesic prematurely. Medical and nursing staff tend to underestimate pain in children and this is borne out by studies of the assessments of pain made by children themselves of their pain experience when compared to the assessments made by parents or staff(RCN, 1999). Many staff still feel that pain can only be reduced but not controlled or prevented.

Practice can be changed by education. This is illustrated by the changes in perception and practice amongst paediatric anaesthetists surveyed in 1988 and again in 1995 (Table 1.5)(De Lima et al., 1996). This highlights very well the evolution of more comprehensive analgesic prescribing and more appropriate use of local anaesthetics, opioids and NSAIDs.

TABLE 1.5: RESULTS OF TWO SURVEYS OF PAEDIATRIC ANAESTHETISTS' PERCEPTIONS AND PRACTICE IN 1995 COMPARED WITH 1988(De Lima et al., 1996)

	1988	1995
% who thought neonates did not feel pain	**13%**	**0%**
% who prescribed opioids for neonates after major surgery	**10%**	**91%**
% who used local anaesthetic block or infiltration in newborns	**27%**	**88%**
% who used local anaesthetic for minor surgery	**27%**	**99%**

Information should be provided for children and families in an appropriate language and in written and verbal forms. Parents may ask about the drugs their child may receive and should be given detailed explanations about the options available. The benefits and risks should be clearly explained. If the child is old enough to be consulted then they can be asked about their preferences and should receive an explanation in a form relevant to their age and development. A specific plan of analgesia can then be tailored to the needs of each individual child(Howard, 1996). If parents are familiar with a particular technique such as patient-controlled analgesia, they can encourage their children to use the technique more appropriately. Clear information should help to decrease the level of anxiety and in turn this reduces the analgesic requirement. Parents can also help with assessment of their child, particularly when the child has a mental handicap or has behavioural or developmental problems. The parent is often best at distinguishing the signs of pain in their child and should be encouraged to communicate with staff so that effective analgesia can be maintained. Although a high proportion of parents are resident with their child in hospital, they are more likely to be confident about leaving their child in the care of others if the child is comfortable. A family centred approach to the care of children is very helpful in encouraging the child back towards their normal environment and level of function(RCPCH, 1997, Walker, 2008).

PLANNING PAIN MANAGEMENT

The main factors to consider when planning individualised pain management(Howard, 1996) are listed in Table 1.6.

TABLE 1.6: FACTORS IN PLANNING PAIN MANAGEMENT

age, maturity, physical status, mental status
severity of illness
medical factors: eg. organ dysfunction, asthma, epilepsy, reflux
surgical factors: eg. extent and nature of surgery
anaesthetic factors: eg. airway abnormality, suitability or contraindication to particular analgesic technique
expected pain severity and duration
pain assessment method and training of assessor
past pain experience
child / parental preferences
psychological factors
medical environment: day case, out-patient, a & e, general ward, HDU, ITU
can minimum monitoring standard be met: nurse dependency, assessment of efficacy, monitoring and management of adverse effects
anticipated pathway to recovery
continuing pain control

So, prevention of pain and good pain control are high priorities when dealing with children. The benefits of pain control techniques, when properly selected and applied, outweigh the risks. Education of children parents and staff improves the success and safety of pain control and to ensure *comprehensive* pain prevention and control requires planning and organisation.

IMPROVEMENTS IN THE EVIDENCE-BASE FOR PAEDIATRIC PAIN MANAGEMENT

Recently the evidence underpinning the management of paediatric pain has been collated and evaluated in a number of evidence-based guidelines and systematic reviews. These are presented by analgesic technique (RCA, 1998, ANZCA, 2005, Ansermino et al., 2003, Playfor et al., 2006, Moiniche et al., 2003) or by surgical or medical procedure(APAGBI, 2008). This allows logical selection of analgesia for an individual child, undergoing a specific procedure in a given clinical setting(Walker et al., 2006). In addition, evidence-based guidelines for procedural sedation of children have been developed in Scotland(SIGN, 2004). These guidelines cover all age groups from neonates to adolescents and settings as diverse as clinic, accident and emergency unit, critical care unit, general ward, operating theatre and postoperative ward. For neonates in particular, a large literature has developed to review analgesic techniques based upon better understanding of the developmental aspects of pain physiology and analgesic pharmacology(Walker, 2008) but also due to better appreciation of the need for good studies in this age group(Anand et al., 2005a).

IMPROVEMENTS IN THE UNDERSTANDING OF DEVELOPMENTAL ASPECTS OF PAIN AND ANALGESIA

Developmental physiology of pain

There have been huge advances in understanding of the development of the pain pathways, their function and the changes in distribution of receptors in early life(Fitzgerald, 2005, Baccei and Fitzgerald, 2006, Walker, 2008). This has in turn helped understanding of the changes in pharmacodynamics of analgesics during development and the short- and long-term consequences of pain in early life (see Table 1.1). In the periphery, repeated noxious stimuli produce local sensitisation eg. after heel-stick blood sampling in pre-term neonates. In the spinal cord, excitatory mechanisms mature earlier than inhibitory mechanisms resulting in generalised, mass responses to stimuli that are not well directed and have a low threshold to trigger them, but yet match the stimulus intensity. These stimuli get through even to the immature cortex (Bartocci et al., 2006)

Developmental pharmacology of analgesics

Greater understanding of the effects of size and developmental stage upon pharmacokinetics and dynamics of analgesics has mainly occurred in the last 10 years and this has resulted in much more logical and accurate dosing in children(Berde and Cairns, 2000, Anderson and Meakin, 2002, Anderson and Holford, 2008). Data on developmental changes in body composition, organ function, plasma protein binding and concentration, and elimination enzyme systems and pathways are now available for most analgesics in common use in children.

Stress response and its control

The importance of the stress response to noxious stimuli has been increasingly recognised in paediatrics for around 20 years (Aynsley-Green et al., 1995, Wolf et al., 1998, Anand et al., 1987, Anand and Aynsley-Green, 1988, Anand et al., 1988, Anand and Carr, 1989, Morton, 1989, Anand et al., 1990, Morton, 1990b, Wolf, 1993, Wolf et al., 1993, Glover and Giannakoulopoulos, 1995, Aynsley-Green, 1996, Wolf, 1997, Bell et al., 2004, Humphreys et al., 2004, Stumpe et al., 2006, Grunau et al., 2005). Amelioration of the stress response to noxious stimuli is beneficial for children especially young infants(Anand et al., 2006, D'Apolito, 2006) and those undergoing major surgery(Bouwmeester et al., 2001, Bozkurt, 2002, Bozkurt et al., 2004, Bozkurt et al., 2003). A common stressor in neonates and children is tracheal intubation and, with the availability of new anaesthetic agents and opioids, the possibility of minimising the stress response to tracheal intubation without the use of muscle relaxants has developed from experience in adult practice(Morton and Hamilton, 1986, Steyn et al., 1994, O'Brien et al., 1998, Robinson et al., 1998, Anand et al., 2005b, Aranda et al., 2005, Lago et al., 2005, McGrath, 2005, D'Apolito, 2006, Dempsey et al., 2006, Milesi et al., 2006, APAGBI, 2008, Welzing and Roth, 2006, Playfor et al., 2006).

CHAPTER 2:

IMPROVING ANALGESIC ASSAYS

2.1 Microassay of analgesics

2.1.1 Watson DG, Su Q, Midgley JM, Doyle E, Morton NS. Analysis of unconjugated morphine, codeine, normorphine and morphine as glucuronides in small volumes of plasma from children. Journal of Pharmaceutical & Biomedical Analysis. 1995 Jan;13(1):27-32.

Abstract

A sensitive method for the analysis of unconjugated morphine, codeine, normorphine and total morphine after hydrolysis of glucuronide conjugates is described. The method was applicable to 50-microliter volumes of plasma. The analytes were converted to heptafluorobutyryl (HFB) derivatives before analysis by gas chromatography-negative ion chemical ionization mass spectrometry. Morphine and codeine were quantified against their [2H3]-isotopomers. Linearity, precision and accuracy were quite acceptable (in the 10(-10)-10(-9) g range), and the absolute limits of detection were < 1 pg.

2.1.2 Oliveira EJ, Watson DG, Morton NS. A simple microanalytical technique for the determination of paracetamol and its main metabolites in blood spots. Journal of Pharmaceutical & Biomedical Analysis. 2002 Jul 31;29(5):803-9.

Abstract

The use of blood spot collection cards is a simple way to obtain specimens for analysis of drugs with a narrow therapeutic window. We describe the development and validation of a microanalytical technique for the determination of paracetamol and its glucuronide and sulphate metabolites from blood spots. The method is based on reversed phase high-performance liquid chromatography with ultraviolet detection. The limit of detection of the method is 600 pg on column for paracetamol. Intra- and inter-day precision of the determination of paracetamol was 7.1 and 3.2% respectively. The small volume of blood required (20 microl), combined with the simplicity of the analytical technique makes this a useful procedure for monitoring paracetamol concentrations. The method was applied to the analysis of blood spots taken from neonates being treated with paracetamol.

Discussion

When these studies were developed, there was interest in reinvestigating existing medicines in children and ethical constraints on the volume of blood sampled from small children for the purposes of research. The aim was to develop accurate microassay methods for analgesics in children (Watson et al., 1995, Stumpe et al., 2006, Oliveira et al., 2002) with a view to applying these techniques to infants and neonates. With highly sensitive and specific assay techniques, it has been possible to measure analgesics and their main metabolites and binding proteins in tiny volumes of plasma and in dried blood spots, the latter from a volume of approximately 8 microlitres of blood.

CHAPTER 3:

IMPROVING LOCAL ANAESTHESIA

3.1 Local anaesthesia to abolish injection pain due to propofol in children

3.1.1 Cameron E, Johnston G, Crofts S, Morton NS. The minimum effective dose of lignocaine to prevent injection pain due to propofol in children. Anaesthesia. 1992 Jul;47(7):604-6.

Abstract

In a single-blind study of 100 children aged 1 to 10 years, the minimum effective dose of lignocaine required to prevent injection pain due to propofol was 0.2 mg/kg when veins on the dorsum of the hand were used. This is more than twice the adult value. We concluded that injection pain should not limit the use of propofol in children if an adequate amount of lignocaine is mixed immediately prior to injection.

Discussion

This simple study was undertaken at a time when propofol was just entering clinical practice in paediatric anaesthesia(Morton et al., 1988). It was recognised that propofol caused injection pain in up 85% of children(Valtonen et al., 1989) and this undoubtedly was limiting the clinical use of propofol in paediatric anaesthesia at that time. In adult practice, lignocaine admixture was shown to be effective(Scott et al., 1988, Stafford et al., 1991) while in a pilot study of 50 unpremedicated children, lignocaine 1mg/kg was found to abolish injection pain in veins on the dorsum of the hand(Morton, 1990a). This dose was chosen empirically and after discussion with the ethics committee, a study was designed to define the minimum effective dose. One hundred children aged 1-10 years were given propofol 3mg/kg with stepwise-reducing doses of lignocaine starting at the empirical high dose of 1mg/kg and, if pain free, successive children received a decrement of dose of 0.1mg/kg . If pain was noted, then an increment of 0.1 mg/kg was used in the next child. Using this "up-and-down" technique, a threshold for effective dosing of lignocaine was defined in children when injecting 1% propofol into the veins on the dorsum of the hand. No child who received 0.2mg/kg or more of added lignocaine experienced pain (Figure 3.1).

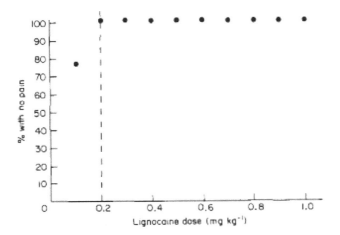

Figure 3.1: The minimum effective dose of lignocaine was found to be 0.2mg/kg for children age 1-10 years when injecting 1% propofol into the veins on the dorsum of the hand.

This minimum effective dose was noted to be approximately twice that of adults (Stafford et al., 1991) and also somewhat higher than the dose described in other paediatric studies at the time which had found unsatisfactory rates of injection pain of 29-60% (Patel et al., 1988, Morton et al., 1988). This study also showed that when injection pain occurred in younger children tended to be more severe.

Clinical implications

This study demonstrated a simple method of abolishing injection pain due to propofol in children and encouraged increased use of propofol by paediatric

34

anaesthetists. Propofol is now routinely used for induction and maintenance of anaesthesia in children(Morton, 2008d, Marsh et al., 1991, Doyle et al., 1993c, Varveris and Morton, 2002, BNFc, 2008, Morton, 1998b, Eyres, 2004, Morton, 2008b).

3.2 Topical local anaesthesia with amethocaine in children

3.2.1 Lawson RA, Smart NG, Gudgeon AC, Morton NS. Evaluation of an amethocaine gel preparation for percutaneous analgesia before venous cannulation in children. British Journal of Anaesthesia. 1995 Sep;75(3):282-5.

We have evaluated the efficacy and safety of a preparation of 4% amethocaine gel in alleviating the pain of venous cannulation in children. In an initial open study of 148 children, clinically acceptable anaesthesia was achieved in 92% of cases. The preparation was then compared with 5% EMLA cream in a single-blind study in 94 patients using an application time of 40 min. We found clinically acceptable conditions in 85% of patients receiving amethocaine gel compared with 66% in the EMLA group. There were no significant adverse effects noted in each group, although 37% of those children treated with amethocaine gel showed localized erythema at the application site. The results suggest that amethocaine gel has greater efficacy and a faster onset time than EMLA cream when used for this purpose in children.

3.2.2 Doyle E, Freeman J, Im NT, Morton NS. An evaluation of a new self-adhesive patch preparation of amethocaine for topical anaesthesia prior to venous cannulation in children. Anaesthesia. 1993 Dec;48(12):1050-2.

Abstract

A new preparation of amethocaine in the form of a self-adhesive patch, designed to provide topical cutaneous anaesthesia prior to venous cannulation, was evaluated in an open study of 189 children. The new preparation of amethocaine was in place for a mean time of 48 min (SD 3.9). Eighty percent of patients had a satisfactory degree of analgesia for venous cannulation. Nine percent of patients experienced moderate pain and 11% experienced severe pain during venous cannulation. In 26% of patients there was slight (24%) or moderate (2%) erythema at the site of application, and in 5% slight oedema was noted at the site of application. Eight percent of patients had slight itching and 1% had moderate itching at the site of application. There was a clinical impression that venous dilatation made cannulation easier than with EMLA cream. These results suggest that this convenient preparation of amethocaine is highly effective at providing adequate topical cutaneous anaesthesia with a short onset time and a low incidence of minor side effects with no evidence of systemic toxicity.

Discussion

Topical local anaesthesia of the skin prior to needling procedures is now

accepted as the standard of care unless there are specific contraindications

(APAGBI, 2008, BNFc, 2008). The evidence is very strong (level A) for effectiveness of these techniques (APAGBI, 2008) and there is now a choice of formulations of various local anaesthetics available (BNFc, 2008). At the time these studies were carried out, only EMLA cream was available in the UK which is an eutectic mixture of lignocaine and prilocaine with an onset time of 40-90 minutes depending on the site of application and the age and ethnicity of the patient (Sweetman, 2007, BNFc, 2008, Freeman et al., 1993). Amethocaine (tetracaine), an ester-local anaesthetic agent, is highly lipophilic with high affinity for neural tissue and seemed therefore to have potential to penetrate intact skin quickly (McCafferty et al., 1989). Early studies showed promising results in adults for venous cannulation (Molodecka et al., 1994) and in children for venepuncture (Woolfson et al., 1990). The onset time appeared to be reliably quicker than EMLA cream, and with a much longer duration of action after removal, probably due to the depot of amethocaine in the stratum corneum (McCafferty et al., 1989). The first study was therefore an open evaluation of a 4% w/w amethocaine gel formulation applied for 40-60 minutes to the dorsum of the hand for venous cannulation in children age 3-12 years (Lawson et al., 1995). The aim was to judge efficacy and safety as a prelude to a comparison with EMLA cream (Lawson et al., 1995). The results showed amethocaine had a quicker onset of action and was more efficacious than EMLA cream after an application time of 40 minutes, although more often produced erythema at the application site.

Amethocaine can also be formulated as a phase-change patch and this had been successfully evaluated in adults (McCafferty and Woolfson, 1993). The self-adhesive patch incorporates a thin film of anhydrous amethocaine base which, upon wetting and reaching body temperature, changes from solid to liquid phase and then more rapidly penetrates intact skin (McCafferty and Woolfson, 1993). This patch applied for an average time of 48 minutes produced satisfactory analgesia for venous cannulation in 80% of children studied with erythema at the application site in about a third of children (Doyle et al., 1993a).

There were no cases of systemic toxicity with these amethocaine formulations which is reassuring for an ester local anaesthetic. Esterases in the skin and blood lead to rapid metabolism with very low plasma concentrations and the depot formed in the stratum corneum results in slow sustained release of the drug thus avoiding high peak plasma concentrations.

These studies were not designed to assess duration of analgesia after removal but amethocaine has been shown to produce several hours of analgesia after removal due to the depot effect noted above (Small et al., 1988).

Clinical implications
Amethocaine gel has been widely adopted for needling procedures in children in the UK since this study was conducted and has a product licence for use in infants and children (Sweetman, 2007, APAGBI, 2008, BNFc, 2008). It has shown particular utility when time is short in day cases and in the emergency or treatment room. The patch formulation has not been released commercially but recently a new lignocaine/amethocaine patch incorporating a thermogenic gel layer has been marketed which shows promise in further speeding onset of analgesia.

3.3 Pharmacokinetics of amide local anaesthetics in children

3.3.1 Doyle E, Morton NS, McNicol LR. Plasma bupivacaine levels after fascia iliaca compartment block with and without adrenaline. Paediatric Anaesthesia. 1997;7(2):121-4.

Abstract

Twenty children undergoing unilateral surgery on the thigh received a fascia iliaca compartment block using 2 mg/kg of bupivacaine with (Group A) or without (Group P) adrenaline 1/200,000. Venous blood samples were taken as 5, 10, 15, 20, 25, 30, 40, 50 and 60 min after injection and assayed for concentrations of bupivacaine. In all subjects an adequate block was produced. Plasma concentrations of bupivacaine in Group P were significantly higher than those in Group A (P < 0.05). The median maximum plasma concentration (Cmax) was 1.1 micrograms/ml (range 0.54-1.29 micrograms/ml) in Group P and 0.35 microgram/ml (range 0.17-0.96 microgram/ml) in Group A. The median time taken to attain Cmax (Tmax) was 20 min (range 10-25 min) in Group P and 45 min (range 5-50 min) in Group A. The median time to first analgesia was 9.75 h (range 3-15 h) in Group P and 10.5 h (range 2.5-21 h) in Group A. The study confirmed the efficacy of the fascia iliaca compartment block in children and showed that when performed with 2 mg/kg of bupivacaine it is associated with plasma concentrations of bupivacaine well within acceptable limits. The addition of adrenaline 1/200,000 to the local anaesthetic solution reduces the maximum plasma concentration reached.

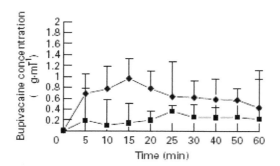

Figure 1
Plasma concentrations (median range) of bupivacaine in Groups P and A. ◆ Plain; ■ Adrenaline.

3.3.2 Hansen TG, Morton NS, Cullen PM, Watson DG. Plasma concentrations and pharmacokinetics of bupivacaine with and without adrenaline following caudal anaesthesia in infants. Acta Anaesthesiologica Scandinavica. 2001 Jan;45(1):42-7.

Abstract

BACKGROUND: The aim of this study was to determine whether the use of adrenaline 1/400000 added to 0.25% bupivacaine significantly delays the systemic absorption of the drug from the caudal epidural space in young infants. METHODS: Fifteen infants less than 5 months of age undergoing minor lower abdominal procedures under a standardised general anaesthetic were randomised to receive a caudal block with either 0.25% plain bupivacaine 2.5 mg/kg (n=7) or bupivacaine 0.25% with 1/400000 adrenaline (n=8). Blood samples were drawn at 30, 60, 90, 180, 240 and 360 min according to the infant's weight and analysed for total and free bupivacaine concentrations using a gas chromatography-mass spectrometry (GC-MS) technique. RESULTS: The total C(MAX) and T(MAX) were comparable in both groups. The total bupivacaine concentration at t=360 min was significantly higher in the "adrenaline" group compared to the "plain" group, i.e. a median (range) 742 ng/ml (372-1423 ng/ml) vs. 400.5 ng/ml (114-446 ng/ml), P=0.0080. The median "apparent" terminal half-life (t1/2) was significantly longer in the "adrenaline" group (363 min; range 238-537 min) compared to the "plain" group (n=6) (165 min; range 104-264 min), P=0.0087. The free bupivacaine concentrations (n=3 in both groups) ranged between 13 ng/ml and 52 ng/ml, corresponding to a percentage of free bupivacaine between 1.3% and 6.7%. CONCLUSION: The addition of 1/400.000 adrenaline prolongs the systemic absorption of caudally administered bupivacaine in infants less than 5 months of age.

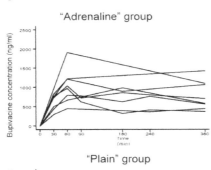

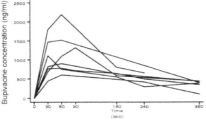

Pharmacokinetic parameters, median (range)		
	Plain group	Adrenaline group
T_{MAX} (min)	60 (30–240)	60 (60–360)
C_{MAX} (ng/ml)	1109 (607–2195)	1012 (449–1909)
K_{el}* (min^{-1})	0.00420 (0.00240–0.00665)	0.00220 (0.00115–0.00291)
$t_{½}$** (min)	165 (104–264) (n=6)	363 (238–537) (n=5)
C_{360}*** (ng/ml)	400.5 (114–446)	742 (372–1423)

* $P=0.00152$
** $P=0.0087$
*** $P=0.0080$.

Discussion

Local anaesthetic techniques are regarded as the foundation of perioperative pain control in children (APAGBI, 2008) and single injection techniques are still the most commonly used (Morton, 1998a, Lonnqvist and Morton, 2005a, Morton, 2007). At the time these studies were conducted, bupivacaine was the usual local anaesthetic agent used in children but of course has been superceded by the new amide local anaesthetic agents, levobupivacaine and ropivacaine (Sweetman, 2007, Morton, 2007, APAGBI, 2008, BNFc, 2008). These studies were designed primarily to assess the plasma concentration-time profiles of bupivacaine in infants and children after caudal or fascia iliaca compartment blocks and the influence of added adrenaline (Doyle et al., 1997, Hansen et al., 2001). Caudal blocks was much studied but the fascia iliaca compartment block was less well known at that time. The study of this block showed safe local anaesthetic plasma concentrations with or without adrenaline and median duration of analgesia of around 10 hours which was not affected by adrenaline. In individual cases much longer analgesia was seen. The caudal study focussed on infants because the effect of adrenaline on plasma concentration-time profiles of bupivacaine had not previously been described. This study confirmed safe plasma concentrations of bupivacaine in this young age group and that 1:400,000 adrenaline prolongs the systemic absorption of caudally administered bupivacaine.

Clinical implications

The addition of vasoconstrictors and other analgesic additives has become commonplace and the evidence of risks and benefits have recently been reviewed (Ansermino et al., 2003, de Beer and Thomas, 2003, APAGBI, 2008, Mazoit and Dalens, 2004). Bupivacaine is known to produce more cardiac and central nervous system toxicity than the new agents levobupivacaine and ropivacaine (Morton, 2004, Rapp et al., 2004, Ivani et al., 2002, Lerman et al., 2003, Taylor et al., 2003, Chalkiadis et al., 2004, De Negri et al., 2004, Ivani et al., 2004, Ivani et al., 1998a, Ivani et al., 1998b, Da Conceicao et al., 1999, Morton, 2000, Stumpe et al., 2000, Bosenberg et al., 2001, Dalens et al., 2001, De Negri et al., 2001a, De Negri et al., 2001b) and despite many years of safe clinical use in infants and children based on clinical studies and pharmacokinetic studies, many clinicians have changed their practice to adopt the new agents for single injection blocks and infusion techniques. It is hard not to agree with this, in particular when there is hardly any cost differential and the new agents are widely available. In infants and in particular neonates, where local anaesthetic toxicity is a real risk, the new agents have superceded bupivacaine.

CHAPTER 4:

IMPROVING OPIOID TECHNIQUES

4.1 Patient-controlled analgesia in children

4.1.1 Irwin M, Gillespie JA, Morton NS. Evaluation of a disposable patient-controlled analgesia device in children.[see comment]. British Journal of Anaesthesia. 1992 Apr;68(4):411-3.

Abstract

A disposable patient-controlled analgesia (PCA) device was evaluated in 20 children after major abdominal, urological and orthopaedic surgery. All patients were given a high dependency level of nursing care in general wards. Efficacy (as assessed by hourly pain scores) was comparable to that achieved in a matched control group of 20 children who used the Graseby PCA system. Safety was confirmed by monitoring arterial oxygen saturation, sedation scores and ventilatory frequency. Morphine consumption was similar with the two techniques, but varied widely between patients. The disposable device has a complementary role to play in the provision of a comprehensive pain relief service for children.

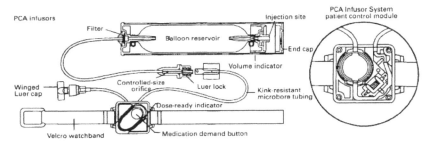

Discussion

At the time this study was published, PCA was not well established in paediatrics.

It was unusual at that time for opioid infusion techniques to be managed in

general postoperative wards and so continuing pain control beyond the early

postoperative period was problematic. A few descriptions of PCA in children had

been published (Rodgers et al., 1988, Schechter et al., 1988, Gaukroger et al.,

1989, Webb et al., 1989, Tyler, 1990, Berde et al., 1991, Gaukroger et al., 1991,

Mackie et al., 1991) but there was a wide variation in regimens and the optimum

regimen had yet to be defined. This study of a disposable device was the first description of its use in children and proved as effective as a conventional electronic PCA pump (Irwin et al., 1992). The department in Glasgow at this time completed a portfolio of studies on PCA in children to try to define the optimum regimen for PCA in children, the limits of its application and the monitoring standards for safe use in general ward environments (Doyle et al., 1993b, Doyle et al., 1993d, Doyle et al., 1994a, Doyle et al., 1994b, Doyle et al., 1994c, Morton and O'Brien, 1999, Munro et al., 2002). From these studies, most of which comprised an MD Thesis for Dr E Doyle, the efficacy and safety of PCA in children from age 5 years of age upwards was established and subsequently confirmed by many other studies (Shapiro et al., 1993, Weldon et al., 1993, Dunbar et al., 1995, Collins et al., 1996, Hansen et al., 1996, Tyler et al., 1996, Kanagasundaram et al., 1997, McNeely and Trentadue, 1997, Petrat et al., 1997, Trentadue et al., 1998, Peters et al., 1999, Sutters et al., 1999, Kotzer and Foster, 2000, Lambert and Mayor, 2000, Bozkurt, 2002, Dix et al., 2003, Jacob et al., 2003, Ozalevli et al., 2005, Kelly et al., 2006).

Clinical implications

PCA is now widely used in children and has a strong body of evidence supporting its safety and effectiveness (ANZCA, 2005, APAGBI, 2008). New features highlighted by the Glasgow studies were the usefulness of a low-dose background infusion in improving sleep patterns, clarification of the monitoring requirements for safe use in general wards, the optimum regimen for paediatric PCA (20 micrograms/kg bolus, 5 minute lockout interval, 4-5 micrograms/kg/h background infusion), the possibilities for anti-emetic treatment, the fact that the Subcutaneous route for PCA worked in children and the usefulness of disposable PCA devices in children.

CHAPTER 5:

IMPROVING USE OF NSAIDS AND PARACETAMOL

4.1 Morphine-sparing effect of NSAIDs and paracetamol in children

4.1.1 Morton NS, O'Brien K. Analgesic efficacy of paracetamol and diclofenac in children receiving PCA morphine. British Journal of Anaesthesia. 1999 May;82(5):715-7.

Abstract

We studied 80 children, aged 5-13 yr, who received PCA with morphine after appendicectomy using a standardized tracheal general anaesthetic. All patients received morphine 0.1 mg/kg before surgical incision and all had wound infiltration with bupivacaine 1 mg/kg at the end of surgery. Patients were allocated randomly to receive postoperative analgesia with PCA morphine alone, morphine plus diclofenac 1 mg/kg, morphine plus paracetamol 15-20 mg/kg or morphine plus a combination of both diclofenac and paracetamol. Cumulative morphine consumption was significantly reduced by concurrent administration of diclofenac but no additive effect of paracetamol was demonstrable with the doses used in the study. Analgesia, as assessed by movement pain scoring, was significantly improved by the addition of diclofenac despite lower morphine consumption. Adverse effects and duration of PCA were comparable in the four groups.

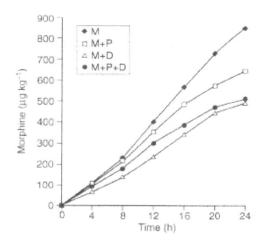

Fig 1 Cumulative morphine use over the first 24 h in group M (morphine alone), group M + P (morphine + paracetamol), group M + D (morphine + diclofenac) and group M + P + D (morphine + paracetamol + diclofenac). Values are mean µg kg^{-1} at 4-hourly intervals. The two groups who received diclofenac had significantly lower morphine consumption at 24 h than the morphine only group ($P < 0.01$).

Discussion

NSAIDs and paracetamol are now well established in paediatric practice (Sweetman, 2007, RCA, 1998, ANZCA, 2005, APAGBI, 2008, BNFc, 2008). The concept of concurrent administration of analgesics from different classes was not accepted in paediatrics at this time however and this study was designed to demonstrate the effectiveness of co-analgesia (Morton and O'Brien, 1999). The results showed that diclofenac produced a 40% morphine-sparing effect and better analgesia while paracetamol produced approximately 20% morphine-sparing. The dose of paracetamol used in this study was low however and recent advice suggests larger doses should be used (Anderson and Palmer, 2006).

Clinical implications

Multimodal co-analgesia is now routinely used and advised for paediatric pain control (APAGBI, 2008, Walker et al., 2006, ANZCA, 2005). The methodology used in this study may be useful in objectively evaluating new NSAIDs and new formulations, such as intravenous paracetamol, in children.

4.2 Pharmacokinetics of paracetamol in children

4.2.1 Hansen TG, O'Brien K, Morton NS, Rasmussen SN. Plasma paracetamol concentrations and pharmacokinetics following rectal administration in neonates and young infants. Acta Anaesthesiologica Scandinavica. 1999 Sep;43(8):855-9.

Abstract

BACKGROUND: Despite widespread use in children pharmacokinetic data about paracetamol are relatively scarce, not the least in the youngest age groups. This study aimed to describe plasma paracetamol concentrations and pharmacokinetics of a single rectal paracetamol dose in neonates and young infants. METHODS: Perioperatively, 17 neonates and infants < or =160 days of age received one rectal paracetamol dose (mean 23.9 mg/kg (+/-4.2 mg/kg)). Blood samples were drawn at 60, 120, 180, 240, 300 and 360 min, according to the infants' weights. Plasma paracetamol concentrations were measured by a Colorometric Assay, Ectachem Clinical Chemistry Slides (Johnson & Johnson Clinical Diagnostics). RESULTS: The plasma paracetamol concentrations were mainly below the therapeutic (i.e. antipyretic) range of 66-132 micromol/l and did not exceed 160 micromol/l in any infant. The mean maximum plasma concentration (Cmax) was 72.4 micromol/l (+/-33.5 micromol/l) and the time to Cmax, i.e. the mean Tmax was 102.4 min (_+59.1 min). The mean "apparent" terminal half-life (n=10) was 243.6 min (+/- 114.1 min). CONCLUSION: The absorption of rectal paracetamol (mean dose 23.9 mg/kg, +/-4.2mg/kg) in young infants <160 days is variable and often prolonged and achieves mainly subtherapeutic plasma concentrations.

Discussion

This study demonstrated the poor bioavailability of suppository formulations of

paracetamol in neonates, infants and children, which is now well established

(Anderson, 1998, Anderson and Holford, 2008). This study was incorporated

into a pooled analysis of paracetamol pharmacokinetics in infants which helped

rationalise dosing regimens (Anderson, 1998, Anderson and Palmer, 2006).

49

CHAPTER 6:

IMPROVING STRESS CONTROL IN CHILDREN

6.1 Reducing the stress response to open heart surgery in children

6.1.1 Laycock GJ, Mitchell IM, Paton RD, Donaghey SF, Logan RW, Morton NS. EEG burst suppression with propofol during cardiopulmonary bypass in children: a study of the haemodynamic, metabolic and endocrine effects. British Journal of Anaesthesia. 1992 Oct;69(4):356-62.

Abstract

We have studied the effects of propofol, given to maintain EEG suppression throughout cardiopulmonary bypass (CPB), in 20 children aged 1-15 yr, in a parallel group comparison. Anaesthesia was produced by fentanyl 50 micrograms /kg, enflurane or halothane and midazolam 0.1 mg /kg at the start of CPB. After randomization, 50% of the children also received propofol during CPB. All children were cooled during CPB (25-28 degrees C) and pump flows (non-pulsatile) were 2.4 litre min-1 m-2, reducing to 1.2-1.6 litre min-1 m-2 during hypothermia. Large rates of infusion of propofol were required to maintain EEG suppression, particularly during rewarming. Compared with control, the propofol group showed significant increases in mixed venous oxygen saturation and significant reductions in systemic oxygen uptake and glucose and cortisol concentrations. There were no differences in triiodothyronine and lactate concentrations, mean arterial pressure during CPB and inotrope requirement after CPB, or in recovery times.

6.1.2 Bell G, Dickson U, Arana A, Robinson D, Marshall C, Morton N. Remifentanil vs fentanyl/morphine for pain and stress control during pediatric cardiac surgery. Paediatric Anaesthesia. 2004 Oct;14(10):856-60.

Abstract

BACKGROUND: Remifentanil is a short acting, potent synthetic opioid that does not accumulate after infusion or repeated bolus doses. It may be rapidly titrated to the requirements of individual patients. Titrated infusion of remifentanil may be able to provide potent analgesia required for pediatric cardiac surgery and obtund the stress response in theater whilst not having the persistent respiratory depression and sedation seen with longer acting opioids. METHODS: Twenty patients were randomized to receive a titrated infusion of remifentanil (0-1 microg x kg(-1) x min(-1)) or a standard dose of fentanyl (30 microg x kg(-1)) prebypass plus morphine (1 mg x kg(-1)) on rewarming. Blood samples for glucose and cortisol were taken at regular intervals from induction through bypass and into the first 24 h of postoperative intensive care. In addition to biochemical indicators of the stress response we recorded baseline hemodynamic parameters and any acute physiological events. RESULTS: Ten patients received morphine, seven received remifentanil. There were no statistically significant differences between the two treatment groups in cortisol measurements, mean arterial pressure or heart rate recordings. In the last time period the remifentanil group had a larger rise in blood glucose concentration (baseline 3.9, rise 3 mmol x l(-1)) than the fentanyl/morphine group (baseline 4.2 rise 1.9 mmol x l(-1)), CI -4.3 to -0.2. CONCLUSIONS: The only significant difference was in glucose in the postbypass time periods. Although statistically significant, this difference is insufficient evidence of increased stress in the remifentanil group. The results show that in the patients studied there was no clinically important difference between the two techniques.

Discussion

The stress response to surgery in children has been of great interest since Anand's early studies 30 years ago highlighted stress control as an issue for neonates, infants and children undergoing major surgery (Anand et al., 1987, Anand and Aynsley-Green, 1988, Anand et al., 1988, Anand and Carr, 1989, Anand et al., 1990). Regional analgesia techniques (Wolf, 1993, Wolf et al., 1993, Wolf et al., 1998) and a variety of opioids (Bouwmeester et al., 2001, Bozkurt, 2002, van Dijk et al., 2002, Bozkurt et al., 2003, Bozkurt et al., 2004, Humphreys et al., 2004)have been studied in detail. Our first study of propofol was unusual in using deep intravenous anaesthesia to manage the stress response to open heart surgery and cardiopulmonary bypass (Laycock et al., 1992). With more sophisticated depth of anaesthesia monitors now available such as BIS and AEP, this technique can be adapted to modern practice and indeed this is now my normal technique for most paediatric cardiac anaesthesia, using TCI propofol and alfentanil with AEP monitoring. The second study used the new ultra-short-acting opioid remifentanil to achieve stress control in a small study (Bell et al., 2004). A number of others have investigated remifentanil in neonates, infants and children (Davis et al., 1999, Hammer et al., 2005, Welzing and Roth, 2006) although there are concerns about acute tolerance (Crawford et al., 2006).

6.2 Stress free tracheal intubation in children without the use of muscle relaxants

6.2.1 Steyn MP, Quinn AM, Gillespie JA, Miller DC, Best CJ, Morton NS. Tracheal intubation without neuromuscular block in children.[see comment]. British Journal of Anaesthesia. 1994 Apr;72(4):403-6.

Abstract

We have studied 80 healthy children, aged 2-14 yr, undergoing adenotonsillectomy in a double-blind, randomized design. Tracheal intubation facilitated by either suxamethonium 1.5 mg /kg or alfentanil 15 micrograms /kg was compared after induction of anaesthesia with propofol 3-4 mg /kg. The quality of tracheal intubation was graded according to the ease of laryngoscopy, position of the vocal cords, coughing, jaw relaxation and movement of limbs. There were no significant differences in the overall assessment of intubating conditions between the two groups, and all children underwent successful tracheal intubation. Fewer patients coughed (P < 0.014) and limb movement was less common (P < 0.007) after tracheal intubation facilitated by suxamethonium. Alfentanil attenuated the haemodynamic responses to tracheal intubation.

6.2.2 Robinson DN, O'Brien K, Kumar R, Morton NS. Tracheal intubation without neuromuscular blockade in children: a comparison of propofol combined either with alfentanil or remifentanil. Paediatric Anaesthesia. 1998;8(6):467-71.

Abstract

Forty healthy children, aged between two and 12 years of age undergoing elective surgery where the anaesthetic technique involved tracheal intubation followed by spontaneous ventilation were studied. Induction of anaesthesia was with either alfentanil 15 micrograms./kg or remifentanil 1 microgram./kg followed by propofol 4 mg./kg to which lignocaine 0.2 mg./kg had been added. Intubating conditions were graded on a four point scale for ease of laryngoscopy, vocal cord position, degree of coughing, jaw relaxation and limb movement. All children were successfully intubated at the first attempt. There were no significant differences in the assessments of intubating conditions between the two groups. Arterial blood pressure and heart changes were similar in the two groups with both alfentanil and remifentanil attenuating the haemodynamic response to tracheal intubation. The time taken to resumption of spontaneous ventilation was similar in both groups.

Discussion

These studies were among the first to explore intubation without muscle

relaxants in children using propofol and short acting opioids (Robinson et al.,

1998, Steyn et al., 1994). Around this time, we also conducted a study comparing the then relatively new agent sevoflurane with halothane for tracheal intubation

(O'Brien et al., 1998). All the studies focussed primarily on the quality of

intubating conditions and the speed of achieving satisfactory conditions. With

the opioid/ propofol techniques it was clear that the stress response related

haemodynamic effects of tracheal intubation were also ameliorated significantly.

CHAPTER 7:

AUDIT, GUIDELINES & PROTOCOLS

Advice to clinicians on assessment and management of pain has been brought together in a number of guidelines in the last 10 years (RCN, 1999, RCA, 1998, ANZCA, 2005, APAGBI, 2008, Playfor et al., 2006, SIGN, 2004). These guidelines cover best practice in procedural analgesia, postoperative analgesia, pain assessment, and sedation and analgesia in paediatric intensive care. Aspects of the implementation of these guidelines has been audited in two major projects covering epidural infusion analgesia (Llewellyn and Moriarty, 2007) in children and opioid infusion techniques in children (Morton, 2008c).

Audit of epidural infusion analgesia

This project involved most of the acute paediatric pain teams throughout the UK and was designed to quantify the risks associated with epidural infusion analgesia in children. Data were collected over five years. 96 incidents were reported in 10,633 epidurals. 56 (1:189) were associated with the insertion or maintenance of the epidural and most were of low severity. 5 incidents were graded as serious (1:2000). Only one child had residual effects (1:10,000). Four incidents of compartment syndrome occurred which were not masked by the epidural. The results of this audit project have been used to produce information for children and families about the risks and benefits of epidural infusion analgesia.

Audit of opioid infusion techniques

Following the success of the National Epidural Audit project, the APAGBI agreed to fund an analogous audit project for opioid infusion techniques in children (continuous infusions, patient-controlled analgesia and nurse-controlled analgesia) (Morton, 2008c). This project is in progress from July 2007-December 2008 and the interim results collated after 6 months reveal 21 reported incidents out of 4273 opioid infusion techniques (1: 200). 9 were graded as severe (1:500) with one child having residual problems at discharge from hospital (1:4273). These serious cases were 1 cardio-respiratory arrest in a neonate, 6 cases of respiratory depression requiring naloxone administration, 2 further cases of respiratory depression requiring bag and mask ventilation and oxygen but no naloxone. A number of less severe opioid-related adverse effects were reported such as pruritis, urinary retention and emesis were reported. These were treated either by stopping the morphine or by switching to another opioid. A number of potential drug calculation and dilution errors were also reported but all were identified before harm occurred. The audit continues until 10,000 cases are registered and this should allow comparison of the relative risks of opioid infusion techniques compared with epidural infusion techniques in children in the UK which, in turn, will help inform families and children in future.

SIGN GUIDELINE 58: SAFE SEDATION OF CHILDREN UNDERGOING DIAGNOSTIC AND THERAPEUTIC PROCEDURES(SIGN, 2004)

This evidence-based guideline was developed by a working group chaired by the author after a Scottish national audit revealed wide variation in paediatric procedural sedation practice across the country (Morton and Oomen, 1998). The guidelines were accompanied by recommendations for consent procedures, monitoring, documentation and case selection (see Appendix 2). Recently, NICE have selected this as a topic for their guidelines programme.

Glasgow Protocol for Acute Pain Management (See Appendix 3)

The local acute pain protocol used in Glasgow is a synthesis of current dosing schedules. This protocol has been developed and evolved since 1994 and has proven to be very successful as a basis for education of doctors and nurses and ensures more equity of pain management across our hospital. Monitoring charts for each technique and pain assessment charting is now routine in the hospital and is regarded as the 6th vital sign. This protocol has informed an RCPCH book on pain management (RCPCH, 1997) and the analgesia section of the British National Formulary for Children (BNFc, 2008).

CHAPTER 8:

CONCLUSIONS

This thesis describes a range of studies that have contributed to improvements in pain management of children over the last 20 years. The focus of most paediatric anaesthetists in the late 1980's was upon immediate anaesthetic management in the operating theatre, with adaptation of new monitoring modalities and general anaesthetic agents to paediatric practice in the interests of safety and improved outcome, especially as sicker and younger infants were subjected to corrective surgery. It was realised that intraoperative regional analgesia and continuing pain control were equally important. The studies described in detail, supplemented by a number of others included in co-worker's theses, have contributed to the evidence base for clinical practice guidelines and protocols which allow extremely successful and safe pain management of the vast majority of children. These techniques have been adopted widely and are now routine practice around the world and can indeed be regarded as the standard of care for children undergoing surgery and diagnostic or therapeutic procedures. The recent collation of evidence-based guidance confirms that pain management of children has improved (APAGBI, 2008, BNFc, 2008, Walker, 2008, ANZCA, 2005).

BIBLIOGRAPHY

ANAND, K. J., VAN DEN ANKER, J. N., BERDE, C. B. & AL, E. (2005a) Analgesia and anesthesia for neonates: study design and ethical issues. *Clinical Therapeutics,* 27, 814-843.

ANAND, K. J. S., ARANDA, J. V., BERDE, C. B., BUCKMAN, S., CAPPARELLI, E. V., CARLO, W., HUMMEL, P., JOHNSTON, C. C., LANTOS, J., TUTAG-LEHR, V., LYNN, A. M., MAXWELL, L. G., OBERLANDER, T. F., RAJU, T. N. K., SORIANO, S. G., TADDIO, A. & WALCO, G. A. (2006) Summary proceedings from the neonatal pain-control group. *Pediatrics,* 117, S9-S22.

ANAND, K. J. S. & AYNSLEY-GREEN, A. (1988) Measuring the severity of surgical stress in neonates. *Journal of Pediatric Surgery,* 23, 297-305.

ANAND, K. J. S. & CARR, D. B. (1989) The neuroanatomy, neurophysilogy, and neurochemistry of pain, stress, and analgesia in newborns and children. *Pediatric Clinics of North America,* 36, 795-822.

ANAND, K. J. S., JOHNSTON, C. C., OBERLANDER, T. F., TADDIO, A., LEHR, V. T. & WALCO, G. A. (2005b) Analgesia and local anesthesia during invasive procedures in the neonate. *Clinical Therapeutics,* 27, 844-76.

ANAND, K. J. S., PHIL, D., HANSEN, D. D. & AL., E. (1990) Hormonal-metabolic stress responses in neonates undergoing cardiac surgery. *Anesthesiology,* 73, 661-670.

ANAND, K. J. S., SIPPEL, W. G. & AYNSLEY-GREEN, A. (1987) Randomized trial of fentanyl anesthesia in preterm neonates undergoing surgery: Effects on stress response. *Lancet,* i, 243-248.

ANAND, K. J. S., SIPPELL, W. G., SCHOFIELD, N. M. & AL., E. (1988) Does halothane anaesthesia decrease the stress response of newborn infants undergoing operation? *British Medical Journal,* 296, 668-672.

ANDERSON, B. J. (1998) What we don't know about paracetamol in children. *Paediatric Anaesthesia,* 8, 451-460.

ANDERSON, B. J. & HOLFORD, N. H. (2008) Mechanism-based concepts of size and maturity in pharmacokinetics. *Annual Reviews of Pharmacology and Toxicology,* 48, 303-332.

ANDERSON, B. J. & MEAKIN, G. H. (2002) Scaling for size: some implications for paediatric anaesthesia dosing. *Paediatr Anaesth,* 12, 205-219.

ANDERSON, B. J. & PALMER, G. M. (2006) Recent developments in the pharmacological management of pain in children. *Current Opinion in Anaesthesiology,* 19, 285-292.

ANSERMINO, M., BASU, R., VANDEBEEK, C. & MONTGOMERY, C. (2003) Nonopioid additives to local anaesthetics for caudal blockade in children: a systematic review. *Paediatr Anaesth.,* 13, 561-573.

ANZCA (2005) Acute Pain Management: Scientific Evidence. 2nd ed. Melbourne.

APAGBI (2008) Good Practice in Postoperative and Procedural Pain. *Pediatric Anesthesia,* 18.

ARANA, A., **MORTON**, N. S. & HANSEN, T. G. (2001) Treatment with paracetamol in infants. *Acta Anaesthesiologica Scandinavica,* 45, 20-9.

ARANDA, J. V., CARLO, W., HUMMEL, P., THOMAS, R., LEHR, V. T. & ANAND, K. J. S. (2005) Analgesia and sedation during mechanical ventilation in neonates. *Clinical Therapeutics,* 27, 877-99.

AYNSLEY-GREEN, A. (1996) Pain and stress in infancy and childhood- where to now? *Paediatr Anaesth,* 6, 167-172.

AYNSLEY-GREEN, A., WARD-PLATT, M. P. & LLOYD-THOMAS, A. R. (1995) Stress and Pain in Infancy and Childhood. *Bailliere's Clinical Paediatrics,* 3, 449-631.

BACCEI, M. & FITZGERALD, M. (2006) Development of pain pathways and mechanisms. IN MCMAHON, S. B. & KOLTZENBURG, M. (Eds.) *Wall and Melzack's Textbook of Pain.* London, Elsevier Churchill Livingstone.

BARTOCCI, M., BERGQVIST, L. L., LAGERCRANTZ, H. & ANAND, K. J. (2006) Pain activates cortical areas in the preterm newborn brain. *Pain,* 122, 109-117.

BELL, G., DICKSON, U., ARANA, A., ROBINSON, D., MARSHALL, C. & **MORTON**, N. (2004) Remifentanil vs fentanyl/morphine for pain and stress control during pediatric cardiac surgery. *Paediatric Anaesthesia,* 14, 856-60.

BERDE, C. B. & CAIRNS, B. (2000) Developmental pharmacology across species: promise and problems. *Anesthesia and Analgesia,* 91, 1-5.

BERDE, C. B., LEHN, B. M., YEE, J. D., SETHNA, N. F. & RUSSO, D. (1991) Patient-controlled analgesia in children and adolescents: a randomized, prospective comparison with intramuscular administration of morphine for postoperative analgesia. *Journal of Pediatrics,* 118, 460-6.

BNFC (2008) *British National Formulary for Children 2008,* London, BMJ Publishing Group Ltd.

BOSENBERG, A. T., THOMAS, J., CRONJE, L., LOPEZ, T., CREAN, P. M., GUSTAFSSON, U., HULEDAL, G. & LARSSON, L. E. (2005) Pharmacokinetics and efficacy of ropivacaine for continuous epidural infusion in neonates and infants. *Paediatric Anaesthesia,* 15, 739-49.

BOSENBERG, A. T., THOMAS, J., LOPEZ, T., HULEDAL, G., JEPPSSON, L. & LARSSON, L. E. (2001) Plasma concentrations of ropivacaine following a single-shot caudal block of 1, 2 or 3 mg/kg in children. *Acta Anaesthesiol Scand.,* 45, 1276-1280.

BOUWMEESTER, N. J., ANAND, K. J., VAN DIJK, M., HOP, W. C., BOOMSMA, F. & TIBBOEL, D. (2001) Hormonal and metabolic stress responses after major surgery in children aged 0-3 years: a double-blind, randomized trial comparing the effects of continuous versus intermittent morphine. *British Journal of Anaesthesia,* 87, 390-9.

BOZKURT, P. (2002) The analgesic efficacy and neuroendocrine response in paediatric patients treated with two analgesic techniques: using morphine-epidural and patient-controlled analgesia. *Paediatric Anaesthesia,* 12, 248-54.

BOZKURT, P., KAYA, G., YEKER, Y., ALTINTA, F., BAKAN, M., HACIBEKIROGLU, M. & BAHAR, M. (2004) Effectiveness of morphine via thoracic epidural vs intravenous infusion on postthoracotomy pain and stress response in children. *Paediatric Anaesthesia,* 14, 748-54.

BOZKURT, P., KAYA, G., YEKER, Y., ALTINTAS, F., BAKAN, M., HACIBEKIROGLU, M. & KAVUNOGLU, G. (2003) Effects of systemic and epidural morphine on antidiuretic hormone levels in children. *Paediatric Anaesthesia,* 13, 508-14.

CAMERON, E., JOHNSTON, G., CROFTS, S. & **MORTON**, N. S. (1992) The minimum effective dose of lignocaine to prevent injection pain due to propofol in children. *Anaesthesia,* 47, 604-6.

CHALKIADIS, G. A., EYRES, R. L., CRANSWICK, N., TAYLOR, R. H. & AUSTIN, S. (2004) Pharmacokinetics of levobupivacaine 0.25% following caudal administration in children under 2 years of age. *Br J Anaesth,* 92, 218-222.

COLLINS, J. J., GEAKE, J., GRIER, H. E., HOUCK, C. S., THALER, H. T., WEINSTEIN, H. J., TWUM-DANSO, N. Y. & BERDE, C. B. (1996) Patient-controlled analgesia for mucositis pain in children: a three-period crossover study comparing morphine and hydromorphone. *Journal of Pediatrics,* 129, 722-8.

CRAWFORD, M. W., HICKEY, C., ZAAROUR, C., HOWARD, A. & NASER, B. (2006) Development of acute opioid tolerance during infusion of remifentanil for pediatric scoliosis surgery. *Anesthesia & Analgesia,* 102, 1662-7.

D'APOLITO, K. C. (2006) State of the science: procedural pain management in the neonate. *Journal of Perinatal & Neonatal Nursing,* 20, 56-61.

DA CONCEICAO, M. J., COELHO, L. & KHALIL, M. (1999) Ropivacaine 0.25 % compared with bupivacaine 0.25 % by the caudal route. *Paediatr Anaesth,* 9, 229-233.

DALENS, B., ECOFFEY, C., JOLY, A., GIAUFRE, E., GUSTAFSSON, U., HULEDAL, G. & LARSSON, L. E. (2001) Pharmacokinetics and analgesic effect of ropivacaine following ilioinguinal/ iliohypogastric nerve block in children. *Paediatr Anaesth,* 11, 415-420.

DAVIS, P. J., WILSON, A. S., SIEWERS, R. D., PIGULA, F. A. & LANDSMAN, I. S. (1999) The effects of cardiopulmonary bypass on remifentanil kinetics in children undergoing atrial septal defect repair. *Anesth Analg,* 89, 904-908.

DE BEER, D. A. & THOMAS, M. L. (2003) Caudal additives in children-solutions or problems? *Br J Anaesth,* 90, 487-498.

DE LIMA, J., LLOYD-THOMAS, A. R., HOWARD, R. F., SUMNER, E. & QUINN, T. M. (1996) Infant and neonatal pain: anaesthetists' perceptions and prescribing patterns. *British Medical Journal,* 313, 787.

DE NEGRI, P., IVANI, G., TIRRI, T., MODANO, P., REATO, C., EKSBORG, S. & LONNQVIST, P. A. (2004) A comparison of epidural bupivacaine, levobupivacaine, and ropivacaine on postoperative analgesia and motor blockade. *Anesth Analg,* 99, 45-48.

DE NEGRI, P., IVANI, G., VISCONTI, C. & DE VIVO, P. (2001a) How to prolong postoperative analgesia after caudal anaesthesia with ropivacaine in children: S-ketamine versus clonidine. *Paediatr Anaesth,* 11, 679-683.

DE NEGRI, P., IVANI, G., VISCONTI, C., DE VIVO, P. & LÖNNQVIST, P. A. (2001b) The dose-response relationship for clonidine added to a postoperative continuous epidural infusion of ropivacaine in children. *Anesth Analg,* 93, 71-76.

DEMPSEY, E. M., AL HAZZANI, F., FAUCHER, D. & BARRINGTON, K. J. (2006) Facilitation of neonatal endotracheal intubation with mivacurium and fentanyl in the neonatal intensive care unit. *Archives of Disease in Childhood Fetal & Neonatal Edition,* 91, F279-82.

DIX, P., MARTINDALE, S. & STODDART, P. A. (2003) Double-blind randomized placebo-controlled trial of the effect of ketamine on postoperative morphine consumption in children following appendicectomy. *Paediatric Anaesthesia,* 13, 422-6.

DOYLE, E., BYERS, G., MCNICOL, L. R. & **MORTON**, N. S. (1994a) Prevention of postoperative nausea and vomiting with transdermal hyoscine in children using patient-controlled analgesia. *British Journal of Anaesthesia,* 72, 72-6.

DOYLE, E., FREEMAN, J., IM, N. T. & **MORTON**, N. S. (1993a) An evaluation of a new self-adhesive patch preparation of amethocaine for topical anaesthesia prior to venous cannulation in children. *Anaesthesia,* 48, 1050-2.

DOYLE, E., HARPER, I. & **MORTON**, N. S. (1993b) Patient-controlled analgesia with low dose background infusions after lower abdominal surgery in children. *British Journal of Anaesthesia,* 71, 818-22.

DOYLE, E., MCFADZEAN, W. & **MORTON**, N. S. (1993c) IV anaesthesia with propofol using a target-controlled infusion system: comparison with inhalation anaesthesia for general surgical procedures in children. *British Journal of Anaesthesia,* 70, 542-5.

DOYLE, E., **MORTON**, N. S. & MCNICOL, L. R. (1994b) Comparison of patient-controlled analgesia in children by i.v. and s.c. routes of administration. *British Journal of Anaesthesia,* 72, 533-6.

DOYLE, E., **MORTON**, N. S. & MCNICOL, L. R. (1997) Plasma bupivacaine levels after fascia iliaca compartment block with and without adrenaline. *Paediatric Anaesthesia,* 7, 121-4.

DOYLE, E., MOTTART, K. J., MARSHALL, C. & **MORTON**, N. S. (1994c) Comparison of different bolus doses of morphine for patient-controlled analgesia in children. *British Journal of Anaesthesia,* 72, 160-3.

DOYLE, E., ROBINSON, D. & **MORTON**, N. S. (1993d) Comparison of patient-controlled analgesia with and without a background infusion after lower abdominal surgery in children. *British Journal of Anaesthesia,* 71, 670-3.

DUNBAR, P. J., BUCKLEY, P., GAVRIN, J. R., SANDERS, J. E. & CHAPMAN, C. R. (1995) Use of patient-controlled analgesia for pain control for children receiving bone marrow transplant. *Journal of Pain & Symptom Management,* 10, 604-11.

EYRES, R. (2004) Update on TIVA. *Paediatric Anaesthesia,* 14, 374-9.

FINLEY, G. A. & MCGRATH, P. J. (2001) *Acute and Procedure Pain in Infants and Children.,* Seattle, IASP Press.

FITZGERALD, M. (2005) The development of nociceptive circuits. *National Review of Neuroscience,* 6, 507-520.

FREEMAN, J. A., DOYLE, E., IM, N. G. T. & **MORTON**, N. S. (1993) Topical anaesthesia of the skin: a review. *Paediatric Anaesthesia,* 3, 129-138.

GAUKROGER, P. B., CHAPMAN, M. J. & DAVEY, R. B. (1991) Pain control in paediatric burns--the use of patient-controlled analgesia. *Burns,* 17, 396-9.

GAUKROGER, P. B., TOMKINS, D. P. & VAN DER WALT, J. H. (1989) Patient-controlled analgesia in children. *Anaesthesia & Intensive Care,* 17, 264-8.

GLOVER, V. & GIANNAKOULOPOULOS, X. (1995) Stress and pain in the fetus. *Baillieres Clinical Paediatrics,* 3, 495-510.

GRUNAU, R. E., HOLSTI, L., HALEY, D. W., OBERLANDER, T., WEINBERG, J., SOLIMANO, A., WHITFIELD, M. F., FITZGERALD, C. & YU, W. (2005) Neonatal procedural pain exposure predicts lower cortisol and behavioral reactivity in preterm infants in the NICU. *Pain,* 113, 293-300.

GRUNAU, R. E., HOLSTI, L. & PETERS, J. W. (2006) Long-term consequences of pain in human neonates. *Seminars in Fetal and Neonatal Medicine,* 11, 268-275.

HAMMER, G. B., RAMAMOORTHY, C., CAO, H., WILLIAMS, G. D., BOLTZ, M. G., KAMRA, K. & DROVER, D. R. (2005) Postoperative analgesia after spinal blockade in infants and children undergoing cardiac surgery. *Anesthesia & Analgesia,* 100, 1283-8.

HANSEN, T. G., HENNEBERG, S. W. & HOLE, P. (1996) Age-related postoperative morphine requirements in children following major surgery--an assessment using patient-controlled analgesia (PCA). *European Journal of Pediatric Surgery,* 6, 29-31.

HANSEN, T. G., **MORTON**, N. S., CULLEN, P. M. & WATSON, D. G. (2001) Plasma concentrations and pharmacokinetics of bupivacaine with and without adrenaline following caudal anaesthesia in infants. *Acta Anaesthesiologica Scandinavica,* 45, 42-7.

HANSEN, T. G., O'BRIEN, K., **MORTON**, N. S. & RASMUSSEN, S. N. (1999) Plasma paracetamol concentrations and pharmacokinetics following rectal administration in neonates and young infants. *Acta Anaesthesiologica Scandinavica,* 43, 855-9.

HARVEY, A. J. & **MORTON**, N. S. (2007) Management of procedural pain in children. *Arch. Dis. Child. Ed. Pract. ,* 92, 20-26.

HERMANN, C., HOHMEISTER, J., DEMIRAKCA, S., ZOHSEL, K. & FLOR, H. (2006) Long-term alteration in pain sensitivity in school-aged children with early pain experiences. *Pain,* 125, 278-285.

HOWARD, R. F. (1996) Planning for pain relief. *Bailliere's Clinical Anaesthesiology,* 10, 657-675.

HUMPHREYS, N., BAYS, S. M. A., PAWADE, A., PARRY, A. & WOLF, A. R. (2004) Prospective randomized controlled trial of high dose opioid vs high spinal anaesthesia in infant heart surgery with cardiopulmonary bypass: effects on stress and inflammation. *Paediatr Anaesth,* 14, 705.

IRWIN, M., GILLESPIE, J. A. & **MORTON**, N. S. (1992) Evaluation of a disposable patient-controlled analgesia device in children.[see comment]. *British Journal of Anaesthesia,* 68, 411-3.

IVANI, G., DE NEGRI, P., LONNQVIST, P. A., L'ERARIO, M., MOSSETTI, V., DIFILIPPO, A. & ROSSO, F. (2004) Caudal anesthesia for minor pediatric surgery: ropivacaine 0.2 % vs. levobupivacaine 0.2 %. *Paediatr Anaesth,* In press.

IVANI, G., DENEGRI, P., CONIO, A., GROSSETTI, R., VITALE, P., VERCELLINO, C., GAGLIARDI, F., EKSBORG, S. & LONNQVIST, P. A. (2002) Comparison of racemic bupivacaine, ropivacaine, and levo-bupivacaine for pediatric caudal anesthesia: effects on postoperative analgesia and motor block. *Reg Anesth Pain Med,* 27, 157-161.

IVANI, G., LAMPUGNANI, E., TORRE, M., CALEVO MARIA, G., DENEGRI, P., BORROMETI, F., MESSERI, A., CALAMANDREI, M., LONNQVIST, P. A. & **MORTON**, N. S. (1998a) Comparison of ropivacaine with bupivacaine for paediatric caudal block. *British Journal of Anaesthesia,* 81, 247-8.

IVANI, G., MERETO, N., LAMGPUGNANI, E., DE NEGRI, P., TORRE, M., MATTIOLOI, G., JASONNI, V. & LONNQVIST, P. A. (1998b) Ropivacaine in paediatric surgery: preliminary results. *Paediatr Anaesth,* 8, 127-130.

JACOB, E., MIASKOWSKI, C., SAVEDRA, M., BEYER, J. E., TREADWELL, M. & STYLES, L. (2003) Management of vaso-occlusive pain in children with sickle cell disease. *Journal of Pediatric Hematology/Oncology,* 25, 307-11.

KANAGASUNDARAM, S. A., COOPER, M. G. & LANE, L. J. (1997) Nurse-controlled analgesia using a patient-controlled analgesia device: an alternative strategy in the management of severe cancer pain in children. *Journal of Paediatrics & Child Health,* 33, 352-5.

KELLY, J. J., DONATH, S., JAMSEN, K. & CHALKIADIS, G. A. (2006) Postoperative sleep disturbance in pediatric patients using patient-controlled devices (PCA). *Paediatric Anaesthesia,* 16, 1051-6.

KOTZER, A. M. & FOSTER, R. (2000) Children's use of PCA following spinal fusion. *Orthopaedic Nursing,* 19, 19-27; quiz 28-30.

LAGO, P., GUADAGNI, A., MERAZZI, D., ANCORA, G., BELLIENI, C. V., CAVAZZA, A. & THE PAIN STUDY GROUP OF THE ITALIAN SOCIETY OF, N. (2005) Pain management in the neonatal intensive care unit: a national survey in Italy.[see comment]. *Paediatric Anaesthesia,* 15, 925-31.

LAMBERT, A. W. & MAYOR, A. (2000) Analgesic requirements for appendicectomy: the differences between adults and children. *Annals of the Royal College of Surgeons of England,* 82, 111-2.

LAWRIE, S. C., FORBES, D. W., AKHTAR, T. M. & **MORTON**, N. S. (1990) Patient-controlled analgesia in children. *Anaesthesia,* 45, 1074-6.

LAWSON, R. A. & **MORTON**, N. S. (1998) Amethocaine gel for percutaneous local anaesthesia. *Hospital Medicine (London),* 59, 564-6.

LAWSON, R. A., SMART, N. G., GUDGEON, A. C. & **MORTON**, N. S. (1995) Evaluation of an amethocaine gel preparation for percutaneous analgesia before venous cannulation in children. *British Journal of Anaesthesia,* 75, 282-5.

LAYCOCK, G. J., MITCHELL, I. M., PATON, R. D., DONAGHEY, S. F., LOGAN, R. W. & **MORTON**, N. S. (1992) EEG burst suppression with propofol during cardiopulmonary bypass in children: a study of the haemodynamic, metabolic and endocrine effects. *British Journal of Anaesthesia,* 69, 356-62.

LERMAN, J., NOLAN, J., EYRES, R., SCHILY, M., STODDART, P., BOLTON, C. M., MAZZEO, F. & WOLF, A. R. (2003) Efficacy, safety, and pharmacokinetics of levobupivacaine with and without fentanyl after continuous epidural infusion in children: a multicenter trial. *Anesthesiology,* 99, 1166-1174.

LLEWELLYN, N. & MORIARTY, A. (2007) The National Pediatric Epidural Audit. *Pediatric Anesthesia,* 17, 520-533.

LLOYD-THOMAS, A. R. & HOWARD, R. F. (1994) A pain service for children. *Paediatr Anaesth,* 4, 3-15.

LONNQVIST, P.-A. & **MORTON**, N. S. (2006) Paediatric day-case anaesthesia and pain control. *Current Opinion in Anaesthesiology,* 19, 617-21.

LONNQVIST, P. A. & **MORTON**, N. S. (2005a) Postoperative analgesia in infants and children. *British Journal of Anaesthesia,* 95, 59-68.

LONNQVIST, P. A. & **MORTON**, N. S. (2005b) Postoperative analgesia in infants and children.[see comment][erratum appears in Br J Anaesth. 2005 Nov;95(5):725]. *British Journal of Anaesthesia,* 95, 59-68.

MACKIE, A. M., CODA, B. C. & HILL, H. F. (1991) Adolescents use patient-controlled analgesia effectively for relief from prolonged oropharyngeal mucositis pain. *Pain,* 46, 265-9.

MARSH, B., WHITE, M., **MORTON**, N. & KENNY, G. N. (1991) Pharmacokinetic model driven infusion of propofol in children.[see comment]. *British Journal of Anaesthesia,* 67, 41-8.

MARSH, B. J., **MORTON**, N. S., WHITE, M. & KENNY, G. N. (1990) A computer controlled infusion of propofol for induction and maintenance of anaesthesia in children. *Canadian Journal of Anaesthesia,* 37, S97.

MAZOIT, J. X. & DALENS, B. J. (2004) Pharmacokinetics of local anaesthetics in infants and children. *Clinical Pharmacokinetics,* 43, 17-32.

MCCAFFERTY, D. F. & WOOLFSON, A. D. (1993) New patch delivery system for percutaneous local anaesthesia. *British Journal of Anaesthesia,* 71, 370-374.

MCCAFFERTY, D. F., WOOLFSON, A. D. & BOSTON, V. (1989) In vivo assessment of percutaneous local anaesthetic preparations. *British Journal of Anaesthesia,* 62, 17-21.

MCGRATH, J. M. (2005) Use of analgesia and sedation for intubation in the neonatal intensive care unit. *Journal of Perinatal & Neonatal Nursing,* 19, 293-4.

MCKENZIE, I., GAUKROGER, P. B., RAGG, P. & BROWN, T. C. K. (1997) *Manual of Acute Pain Management in Children.,* London, Churchill Livingstone.

MCNEELY, J. K. & TRENTADUE, N. C. (1997) Comparison of patient-controlled analgesia with and without nighttime morphine infusion following lower extremity surgery in children. *Journal of Pain & Symptom Management,* 13, 268-73.

MILESI, C., PIDOUX, O., SABATIER, E., BADR, M., CAMBONIE, G. & PICAUD, J. C. (2006) Nitrous oxide analgesia for intubating preterm neonates: a pilot study. *Acta Paediatrica,* 95, 1104-8.

MOINICHE, S., ROMSING, J., DAHL, J. & TRAMER, M. R. (2003) Nonsteroidal antiinflammatory drugs and the risk of operative site bleeding after tonsillectomy: a quantitative systematic review. *Anesth Analg,* 96, 68-77.

MOLODECKA, J., STENHOUSE, C., JONES, J. M. & TOMLINSON, A. (1994) Comparison of percutaneous anaesthesia for venous cannulation after topical application of either amethocaine or EMLA cream. *British Journal of Anaesthesia,* 72, 174-176.

MORTON, N. (1993) Managing pain in children. Balanced analgesia for children. *Nursing Standard,* 7, 8-10.

MORTON, N. S. (1989) Pulmonary surfactant: physiology, pharmacology and clinical uses. *British Journal of Hospital Medicine,* 42, 52-8.

MORTON, N. S. (1990a) Abolition of injection pain due to propofol in children. *Anaesthesia,* 45, 70.

MORTON, N. S. (1990b) Exogenous surfactant treatment for the adult respiratory distress syndrome? A historical perspective. *Thorax,* 45, 825-30.

MORTON, N. S. (1998a) *Acute Paediatric Pain Management - a practical guide.,* London, WB Saunders.

MORTON, N. S. (1998b) Total intravenous anaesthesia (TIVA) in paediatrics: advantages and disadvantages.[see comment]. *Paediatric Anaesthesia,* 8, 189-94.

MORTON, N. S. (2000) Ropivacaine in children. *British Journal of Anaesthesia,* 85, 344-6.

MORTON, N. S. (2004) Local and regional anaesthesia in infants. *Continuing Education in Anaesthesia, Critical Care and Pain,* 4, 148-151.

MORTON, N. S. (2007) Management of postoperative pain in children. *Arch. Dis. Child. Ed. Pract.,* 92, 14-19.

MORTON, N. S. (2008a) Acute Pain Relief Service Protocol. Glasgow, Royal Hospital for Sick Children.

MORTON, N. S. (2008b) Intravenous anaesthetic agents. IN SURY, M., BINGHAM, R. & LLOYD-THOMAS, A. R. (Eds.) *Hatch & Sumner's Paediatric Anaesthesia.* 3rd ed. London, Arnold.

MORTON, N. S. (2008c) National Audit of Opioid Infusion Techniques in Children. *Pediatric Anesthesia,* (In press).

MORTON, N. S. (2008d) Total Intravenous Anesthesia. IN COTE, C. J., LERMAN, J. & TODRES, I. D. (Eds.) *A Practice of Anesthesia for Infants and Children.* 4th ed. Boston, Elsevier.

MORTON, N. S., BENHAM, S. W., LAWSON, R. A. & MCNICOL, L. R. (1997) Diclofenac vs oxybuprocaine eyedrops for analgesia in paediatric strabismus surgery. *Paediatric Anaesthesia,* 7, 221-6.

MORTON, N. S. & HAMILTON, W. F. (1986) Alfentanil in an anaesthetic technique for penetrating eye injuries. *Anaesthesia,* 41, 1148-51.

MORTON, N. S. & O'BRIEN, K. (1999) Analgesic efficacy of paracetamol and diclofenac in children receiving PCA morphine.[see comment]. *British Journal of Anaesthesia,* 82, 715-7.

MORTON, N. S. & OOMEN, G. J. (1998) Development of a selection and monitoring protocol for safe sedation of children. *Paediatric Anaesthesia,* 8, 65-8.

MORTON, N. S., WEE, M., CHRISTIE, G., GRAY, I. G. & GRANT, I. S. (1988) Propofol for induction of anaesthesia in children. A comparison with thiopentone and halothane inhalational induction. *Anaesthesia,* 43, 350-5.

MUNRO, F. J., FISHER, S., DICKSON, U. & MORTON, N. (2002) The addition of antiemetics to the morphine solution in patient controlled analgesia syringes used by children after an appendicectomy does not reduce the incidence of postoperative nausea and vomiting. *Paediatric Anaesthesia,* 12, 600-3.

NOTCUTT, W. G. (1997) What makes acute pain chronic? *Current Anaesthesia and Critical Care,* 8, 55-61.

O'BRIEN, K., KUMAR, R. & MORTON, N. S. (1998) Sevoflurane compared with halothane for tracheal intubation in children. *British Journal of Anaesthesia,* 80, 452-5.

OLIVEIRA, E. J., WATSON, D. G. & MORTON, N. S. (2002) A simple microanalytical technique for the determination of paracetamol and its main metabolites in blood spots. *Journal of Pharmaceutical & Biomedical Analysis,* 29, 803-9.

OTTANI, A., LEONE, S., SANDRINI, M., FERRARI, A. & BERTOLINI, A. (2006) The analgesic activity of paracetamol is prevented by the blockade of cannabinoid CB1 receptors. *European Journal of Pharmacology,* 531, 280-281.

OZALEVLI, M., UNLUGENC, H., TUNCER, U., GUNE, Y. & OZCENGIZ, D. (2005) Comparison of morphine and tramadol by patient-controlled analgesia for postoperative analgesia after tonsillectomy in children. *Paediatric Anaesthesia,* 15, 979-84.

PATEL, D. K., KEELING, P. A., NEWMAN, G. B. & RADFORD, P. (1988) Induction dose of propofol in children. *Anaesthesia,* 43, 949-952.

PETERS, J. W., BANDELL HOEKSTRA, I. E., HUIJER ABU-SAAD, H., BOUWMEESTER, J., MEURSING, A. E. & TIBBOEL, D. (1999) Patient controlled analgesia in children and adolescents: a randomized controlled trial. *Paediatric Anaesthesia,* 9, 235-41.

PETERS, J. W., SCHOUW, R., ANAND, K. J., VAN DIJK, M., DUIVENVOORDEN, H. J. & TIBBOEL, D. (2005) Does neonatal surgery lead to increased pain sensitivity in later childhood? *Pain,* 114, 444-454.

PETRAT, G., KLEIN, U. & MEISSNER, W. (1997) On-demand analgesia with piritramide in children. A study on dosage specification and safety. *European Journal of Pediatric Surgery,* 7, 38-41.

PICKERING, G., LORIOT, M.-A., LIBERT, F., ESCHALIER, A., BEAUNE, P. & DUBRAY, C. (2006) Analgesic effect of acetamonophen in humans: first evidence of a central serotonergic mechanism. *Clinical Pharmacology and Therapeutics,* 79, 371-378.

PLAYFOR, S., JENKINS, I., BOYLES, C., CHOONARA, I., DAVIES, G., HAYWOOD, T., HINSON, G., MAYER, A., **MORTON**, N., RALPH, T. & WOLF, A. (2006) Consensus guidelines on sedation and analgesia in critically ill children. *Intensive Care Medicine,* 32, 1125-36.

RAPP, H.-J., MOLNAR, V., AUSTIN, S., KROHN, S., GADEKE, V., MOTSCH, J., BOOS, K., WILLIAMS, D. G., GUSTAFSSON, U., HULEDAL, G. & LARSSON, L. E. (2004) Ropivacaine in neonates and infants: a population pharmacokinetic evaluation following single caudal block.[see comment]. *Paediatric Anaesthesia,* 14, 724-32.

RCA (1998) Guidelines for the use of non-steroidal anti-inflammatory drugs in the perioperative period. London, Royal College of Anaesthetists.

RCN (1999) Clinical guidelines for the recognition and assessment of acute pain in children. London, Royal College of Nursing.

RCPCH (1997) *Prevention and Control of Pain in Children.,* London, BMJ Publishing Group.

ROBINSON, D. N., O'BRIEN, K., KUMAR, R. & **MORTON**, N. S. (1998) Tracheal intubation without neuromuscular blockade in children: a comparison of propofol combined either with alfentanil or remifentanil. *Paediatric Anaesthesia,* 8, 467-71.

RODGERS, B. M., WEBB, C. J., STERGIOS, D. & NEWMAN, B. M. (1988) Patient-controlled analgesia in pediatric surgery. *Journal of Pediatric Surgery,* 23, 259-62.

RUNCIE, C. J., MACKENZIE, S. J., ARTHUR, D. S. & **MORTON**, N. S. (1993) Comparison of recovery from anaesthesia induced in children with either propofol or thiopentone. *British Journal of Anaesthesia,* 70, 192-5.

SCHECHTER, N. L., BERRIEN, F. B. & KATZ, S. M. (1988) PCA for adolescents in sickle-cell crisis. *American Journal of Nursing,* 88, 719.

SCHMELZLE-LUBIECKI, B. M., CAMPBELL, K. A., HOWARD, R. H., FRANCK, L. & FITZGERALD, M. (2007) Long-term consequences of early infant injury and trauma upon somatosensory processing. *European Journal of Pain,* 11, 799-809.

SCOTT, R. P. F., SAUNDERS, D. A. & NORMAN, J. (1988) Propofol: clinical strategies for preventing the pain on injection. *Anaesthesia,* 43, 492-494.

SHAPIRO, B. S., COHEN, D. E. & HOWE, C. J. (1993) Patient-controlled analgesia for sickle-cell-related pain. *Journal of Pain & Symptom Management,* 8, 22-8.

SIGN (2004) Safe sedation of children undergoing diagnostic and therapeutic procedures. A national clinical guideline.

SMALL, J., WALLACE, R. G., MILLAR, R., WOOLFSON, A. D. & MCCAFFERTY, D. F. (1988) Pain free cutting of split skin grafts by application of percutaneous local anaesthetic cream. *British Journal of Plastic Surgery,* 41, 539-543.

STAFFORD, M. A., HULL, C. J. & WAGSTAFF, A. (1991) Effect of lignocaine on pain during injection of propofol. *British Journal of Anaesthesia,* 66, 406-407P.

STEYN, M. P., QUINN, A. M., GILLESPIE, J. A., MILLER, D. C., BEST, C. J. & **MORTON**, N. S. (1994) Tracheal intubation without neuromuscular block in children.[see comment]. *British Journal of Anaesthesia,* 72, 403-6.

STUMPE, M., MILLER, C., **MORTON**, N. S., BELL, G. & WATSON, D. G. (2006) High-performance liquid chromatography determination of alpha1-acid glycoprotein in small volumes of plasma from neonates. *Journal of Chromatography B: Analytical Technologies in the Biomedical & Life Sciences,* 831, 81-4.

STUMPE, M., **MORTON**, N. S. & WATSON, D. G. (2000) Determination of free concentrations of ropivacaine and bupivacaine in plasma from neonates using small-scale equilibrium-dialysis followed by liquid chromatography-mass spectrometry. *Journal of Chromatography B, Biomedical Sciences & Applications,* 748, 321-30.

SUTTERS, K. A., SHAW, B. A., GERARDI, J. A. & HEBERT, D. (1999) Comparison of morphine patient-controlled analgesia with and without ketorolac for postoperative analgesia in pediatric orthopedic surgery. *American Journal of Orthopedics (Chatham, Nj),* 28, 351-8.

SWEETMAN, S. (2007) *Martindale:the complete drug reference.,* London, Pharmaceutical Press.

TADDIO, A., KATZ, J., ILERSICH, A. L. & AL, E. (1997) Effect of neonatal circumcision on pain response during subsequent routine vaccination. *Lancet,* 349, 599-603.

TAYLOR, R., EYRES, R., CHALKIADIS, G. A. & AUSTIN, S. (2003) Efficacy and safety of caudal injection of levobupivacaine 0.25% in children under 2 years of age undergoing inguinal hernia repair, circumcision or orchidopexy. *Paediatr Anaesth,* 13, 114-121.

TRENTADUE, N. O., KACHOYEANOS, M. K. & LEA, G. (1998) A comparison of two regimens of patient-controlled analgesia for children with sickle cell disease. *Journal of Pediatric Nursing,* 13, 15-9.

TYLER, D. C. (1990) Patient-controlled analgesia in adolescents. *Journal of Adolescent Health Care,* 11, 154-8.

TYLER, D. C., POMIETTO, M. & WOMACK, W. (1996) Variation in opioid use during PCA in adolescents.[see comment]. *Paediatric Anaesthesia,* 6, 33-8.

VALTONEN, M., IISALO, E., KANTO, J. & TIKKANEN, J. (1989) Propofol as an induction agent in children: pain on injection and pharmacokinetics. *Acta Anaesthesiol Scand.,* 33, 152-155.

VAN DIJK, M., BOUWMEESTER, N. J., DUIVENVOORDEN, H. J., KOOT, H. M., TIBBOEL, D., PASSCHIER, J. & DE BOER, J. B. (2002) Efficacy of continuous versus intermittent morphine administration after major surgery in 0-3-

71

year-old infants; a double-blind randomized controlled trial. *Pain,* 98, 305-13.

VARVERIS, D. A. & **MORTON**, N. S. (2002) Target controlled infusion of propofol for induction and maintenance of anaesthesia using the paedfusor: an open pilot study. *Paediatric Anaesthesia,* 12, 589-93.

WALCO, G. A., CASSIDY, R. C. & SCHECHTER, N. L. (1994) Pain, hurt and harm. The ethics of pain control in infants and children. *New England Journal of Medicine,* 331, 541-544.

WALKER, S. M. (2008) Pain in children: recent advances and ongoing challenges. *British Journal of Anaesthesia,* 101, 101-110.

WALKER, S. M., MACINTYRE, P. E., VISSER, E. & SCOTT, D. (2006) Acute pain management: current best evidence provides guide for improved practice. *Pain Medicine,* 7, 3-5.

WATSON, D. G., SU, Q., MIDGLEY, J. M., DOYLE, E. & **MORTON**, N. S. (1995) Analysis of unconjugated morphine, codeine, normorphine and morphine as glucuronides in small volumes of plasma from children. *Journal of Pharmaceutical & Biomedical Analysis,* 13, 27-32.

WEBB, C. J., STERGIOS, D. A. & RODGERS, B. M. (1989) Patient-controlled analgesia as postoperative pain treatment for children. *Journal of Pediatric Nursing,* 4, 162-71.

WELDON, B. C., CONNOR, M. & WHITE, P. F. (1993) Pediatric PCA: the role of concurrent opioid infusions and nurse-controlled analgesia. *Clinical Journal of Pain,* 9, 26-33.

WELZING, L. & ROTH, B. (2006) Experience with remifentanil in neonates and infants. *Drugs,* 66, 1339-50.

WOLF, A. (1993) Treat the babies, not their stress responses. *Lancet,* 342, 324-327.

WOLF, A. (1997) Development of pain and stress responses. IN DALENS, B., MURAT, I. & BUSH, G. (Eds.) *4th European Congress of Paediatric Anaesthesia.* Paris, ADARPEF, FEAPA.

WOLF, A. R., DOYLE, E. & THOMAS, E. (1998) Modifying infant stress responses to major surgery: spinal vs extradural vs opioid analgesia. *Paediatr Anaesth,* 8, 305-311.

WOLF, A. R., EYRES, R. L., LAUSSEN, P. C., EDWARDS, J., STANLEY, I. J., ROWE, P. & SIMON, L. (1993) Effect of extradural analgesia on stress responses to abdominal surgery in infants. *Br J Anaesth,* 70, 654-660.

WOOLFSON, A. D., MCCAFFERTY, D. F. & BOSTON, V. (1990) Clinical experiences with a novel percutaneous amethocaine preparation: prevention of pain due to venepuncture in children. *British Journal of Clinical Pharmacology,* 30, 273-279.

APPENDIX 1:

COPIES OF INDEX PUBLISHED PAPERS WITH COPYRIGHT PERMISSION ARE INCLUDED.

THE FOLLOWING PAPERS ARE AVAILABLE VIA THE FOLLOWING LINK:

http://bja.oxfordjournals.org/

Lawson RA, Smart NG, Gudgeon AC, Morton NS. Evaluation of an amethocaine gel preparation for percutaneous analgesia before venous cannulation in children. British Journal of Anaesthesia. 1995 Sep;75(3):282-5.

Irwin M, Gillespie JA, Morton NS. Evaluation of a disposable patient-controlled analgesia device in children. British Journal of Anaesthesia. 1992 Apr;68(4):411-3.

Morton NS, O'Brien K. Analgesic efficacy of paracetamol and diclofenac in children receiving PCA morphine. British Journal of Anaesthesia. 1999 May;82(5):715-7.

Laycock GJ, Mitchell IM, Paton RD, Donaghey SF, Logan RW, Morton NS. EEG burst suppression with propofol during cardiopulmonary bypass in children: a study of the haemodynamic, metabolic and endocrine effects. British Journal of Anaesthesia. 1992 Oct;69(4):356-62.

Steyn MP, Quinn AM, Gillespie JA, Miller DC, Best CJ, Morton NS. Tracheal intubation without neuromuscular block in children. British Journal of Anaesthesia. 1994 Apr;72(4):403-6.

APPENDIX 3:

ACUTE PAIN PROTOCOL, GLASGOW

ACUTE PAIN RELIEF SERVICE (APRS) PROTOCOL v12.1
October 2006

Minimum monitoring standard

One nurse per 4 patients; continuous pulse oximetry; hourly nurse recordings using appropriate monitoring charts; twice daily visits by pain relief nurse specialist and/or duty anaesthetists; once daily visit by pain consultant.

General points

Doses are a guide only and should be titrated against monitoring results. The medical condition, surgical condition, age and maturity of the child will affect the regimen. If possible ward medical staff should perform refilling of opioid syringes after appropriate training. Programming or reprogramming of PCA devices or epidural pumps should **only** be performed by the APRS. Anaesthetic staff **only** should perform refilling local anaesthetic syringes and epidural top-ups. Ensure all syringes for opioid or local anaesthetic infusions are correctly labelled. Ensure prescription is correctly and legibly written, signed, dated and timed on the additive label, in the drug Kardex and on the monitoring chart. Ensure the appropriate monitoring chart has all the requested information accurately filled in and accompanies the patient to the ward or PICU.

Beware!

Double check: All opioid and local anaesthetic infusions should be checked by 2 practitioners. Check drug dosages, drug dilutions, pump settings, concurrent prescription of different opioids, gravity free flow/ siphonage/ reflux of opioids, injection or infusion of the wrong substance into epidurals.

OPIOIDS

TITRATION TO ANALGESIA WITH IV MORPHINE [ensure appropriate monitoring and availability of naloxone]

Pre-term neonate: give increments of 0.005mg/kg ie. 5micrograms/kg at 5 minute intervals up to 0.025mg/kg ie. 25micrograms/kg

Term neonate: give increments of 0.02mg/kg ie. 20micrograms/kg at 5 minute intervals up to 0.1mg/kg ie. 100micrograms/kg

Age 1-3m: give increments of 0.02mg/kg ie. 20micrograms/kg at 5 minute intervals up to 0.1mg/kg ie. 100micrograms/kg

>3m: give increments of 0.05mg/kg ie. 50micrograms/kg at 5 minute intervals up to 0.1-0.2mg/kg ie. 100-200micrograms/kg

OPIOID INFUSIONS

Loading doses

Consider loading dose of morphine if >3m old give increments of 0.05mg/kg ie. 50micrograms/kg at 5 minute intervals up to 0.1-0.2mg/kg ie. 100-200micrograms/kg; omit if <3m or has good local/ regional block or has received loading dose of morphine or another opioid.

Intravenous morphine infusion (IVM)

Use anti-free flow valve & dedicated cannula if possible. If morphine infusion has to be given concurrently with another infusion use anti-free flow + anti-reflux valves.

Morphine 1mg/kg in 50mls 0.9%saline (≡0.02mg/kg/ml ie.20micrograms/kg/ml); maximum 50mg in 50mls

---

Initial IVM settings for paediatrics

Self-ventilating

Age   Pre-term: up to 0.005mg/kg/h ie. 5micrograms/kg/h ≡ 0.25ml/h

Term neonate: up to 0.08mg/kg/h ie. 8micrograms/kg/h ≡ 0.4ml/h

1-3m: up to 0.010mg/kg/h ie. 10micrograms/kg/h ≡ 0.5ml/h

>3m: up to 0.020mg/kg/h ie. 20micrograms/kg/h ≡ 1ml/h

Ventilated in intensive care

Up to 0.040mg/kg/h ie. 40micrograms/kg/h ≡ 2ml/h

Patient controlled analgesia with morphine (PCAM)

Use anti-free flow valve & dedicated cannula if possible. If morphine infusion has to be given concurrently with another infusion use anti-free flow + anti-reflux valves.

Morphine 1mg/kg in 50mls 0.9%saline ($\equiv$0.02mg/kg/ml ie.20micrograms/kg/ml); maximum 50mg in 50mls (1mg/ml)

Initial IVPCAM settings (20,5,4)

Bolus dose 0.020mg/kg ie. 20micrograms/kg $\equiv$ 1.0ml

maximum bolus dose 1mg (for 50kg+)

Lockout interval 5 minutes

Background infusion 0.004mg/kg/h ie.4micrograms/kg/h $\equiv$ 0.2ml/h [useful in first 24h to improve sleep pattern] *Omit if 50kg+ or if has had single shot epidural or regional block*

Nurse-controlled analgesia with morphine (NCAM)

Use anti-free flow valve. Use dedicated cannula where possible. If morphine infusion has to be given concurrently with another infusion use anti-free flow + antireflux valves.

Morphine 1mg/kg in 50mls 0.9%saline (≡0.02mg/kg/ml
ie.20micrograms/kg/ml); maximum 50mg in 50mls (1mg/ml)

Initial NCAM settings (20,20,20)

Age <1m self-ventilating

Bolus dose 0.005mg/kg ie. 5 micrograms/kg = 0.25ml

Lockout interval 30 minutes

No background infusion

Age 1-3m self-ventilating

Bolus dose 0.010mg/kg ie. 10micrograms/kg ≡ 0.5mlLockout interval 30 minutes

No background infusion

Age > 3m self-ventilating, any age ventilated in intensive care

Bolus dose 0.020mg/kg ie. 20micrograms/kg ≡ 1.0ml

maximum bolus dose 1mg (for 50kg+)

Lockout interval 20 minutes

Background infusion 0.020mg/kg/h ie.20micrograms/kg/h ≡ 1ml/h

---

CO-ANALGESIA FOR ACUTE PAIN

Paracetamol dose as per table below; time the doses for the first 48h; *caution if liver dysfunction, reduce loading dose and increase dosing interval in neonates.*

Oral /rectal route

Age	Oral		Rectal		Maximum daily dose (Oral or rectal)	Duration at max. dose
	Loading dose	Maintenance dose	Loading Dose	Maintenance dose		
Preterm 28-32w	20mg/kg	15mg/kg up to 12hrly	20mg/kg	15mg/kg up to 12hrly	35mg/kg/day	48h
Preterm 32-38w	20mg/kg	20mg/kg up to 8hrly	30mg/kg	20mg/kg up to 12hrly	60mg/kg/day	48h
0-3m	20mg/kg	20mg/kg up to 8hrly	30mg/kg	20mg/kg up to 12hrly	60mg/kg/day	48h
>3m	20mg/kg	15mg/kg up to 4hrly	40mg/kg	20mg/kg up to 6hrly	90mg/kg/day	72h

IV route

Age	IV		Maximum daily dose	Duration at max. dose
	Loading dose	Maintenance dose		
Preterm 28-32w	15mg/kg	15mg/kg up to 12hrly	35mg/kg/day	48h
Preterm 32-38w	15mg/kg	15mg/kg up to 8hrly	45mg/kg/day	48h
0-3m	15mg/kg	15mg/kg up to 8hrly	45mg/kg/day	48h
>3m	15mg/kg	15mg/kg up to 6hrly	60mg/kg/day	72h

Diclofenac Age 6m+: 1mg/kg up to 8hourly o/pr (max 3mg/kg/day or 150mg/day whichever is less) [time doses for first 48h]. *Caution if bleeding risk, asthma, atopy, renal dysfunction, GI ulceration/ bleeding, on anticoagulants, **avoid if <6m.***

Ibuprofen Age 1-3m: 5mg/kg up to 6 hourly oral; **age 3m+:** 10mg/kg up to 8 hourly oral (max. 30mg/kg/day or 2.4g/day whichever is less) [time doses for first 48h]. *Caution if bleeding risk, asthma, atopy, renal dysfunction, GI ulceration/ bleeding, on anticoagulants, **avoid if <1m.***

WEANING FROM COMPLEX ANALGESIA

Ensure adequate doses of co-analgesics are prescribed and are being given to achieve morphine-sparing effect; wean down infusion rate depending on monitoring results; liaise with surgical colleagues about oral intake, rectal route for drugs, mobilisation, dressings, drain/catheter removal. If prolonged opioid use (>5 days) wean slowly (20% per day) to avoid withdrawal syndrome.

For specific cases consider step across analgesia with oro-morph 0.3 mg/kg orally or dihydrocodeine, 0.5-1mg/kg orally 6hourly and ensure parenteral morphine has been stopped (*avoid concurrent prescription of opioids*).

ANTAGONISTS

Use Basic Life Support measures (ABC); give oxygen

For opioid antagonism: Naloxone 2-10micrograms/kg iv stat; can be repeated every 60 seconds or start infusion at 10micrograms/kg/h; use lowest effective dose; if no venous access give IM 100micrograms/kg

For benzodiazepine antagonism: Flumazenil 5micrograms/kg iv stat; can be repeated every 60 seconds or start infusion at 10micrograms/kg/h

Beware seizures precipitated by antagonists.

ANTIEMETICS

Ondansetron 0.1mg/kg (100micrograms/kg) iv or oral; trimeprazine 0.25mg/kg (250micrograms/kg) oral; cyclizine 1mg/kg iv or oral

MUSCLE SPASMS IN ORTHOPAEDICS/ BLADDER SPASMS IN UROLOGY
Diazepam 0.1mg/kg (100micrograms/kg) 6hourly oral

Midazolam infusion 0.025mg/kg/h (25micrograms/kg/h) iv *(ie. ¼ of the sedative dose)* [ensure appropriate monitoring].

DRESSINGS & DRAIN REMOVALS

Consider Entonox (use Entonox protocol), opioid bolus, epidural top up. [ensure appropriate monitoring]

SKIN GRAFT DONOR SITES

Lyofoam dressing soaked with 2mg/kg levobupivacaine, 2.5mg/ml (0.25%) plain/1:200,000 adrenaline; put epidural catheter on dressing surface and infuse levobupivacaine, 2.5mg/ml (0.25%) at 0.1-0.2ml/kg/h ≡ 0.25-0.5mg/kg/h ≡ 250-500micrograms/kg/h; use wound perfusion monitoring chart.

BONE GRAFT DONOR SITES

Wound perfusion with levobupivacaine, 2.5mg/ml (0.25%) plain @ 0.1ml/kg/h ≡ 0.25mg/kg/h ≡ 250micrograms/kg/h; use wound perfusion monitoring chart

EPIDURAL LEVOBUPIVACAINE (PLAIN SOLUTIONS)

In theatre

<8y levobupivacaine, 2.5mg/ml (0.25%) 0.25% up to 1.0ml/kg in fractionated doses (may need 50% less for thoracic epidural)

8y+ levobupivacaine, 5mg/ml (0.5%) up to 0.5ml/kg in fractionated doses (may need 50% less for thoracic epidural)

If <6m use IV route for rescue analgesia and following instructions above for titration to analgesia with IV morphine.

If 6m+ place SC cannula for rescue analgesia and prescribe 0.1mg/kg (100micrograms/kg) sc morphine which can be given by ward nursing staff or ward doctor. If no sc cannula, iv morphine up to 0.1mg/kg (100micrograms/kg) can be given by ward doctor, anaesthetist or certificated nurse following instructions above for titration to analgesia with IV morphine.

In recovery

Check block, check adequacy of analgesia, check adequacy of sedation, check for restlessness.

Top up if required with levobupivacaine, 2.5mg/ml (0.25%), 3.75mg/ml (0.375%) or 5mg/ml (0.5%) as appropriate.

If restless, follow instructions above for titration to analgesia with IV morphine.

If epidural is not working after top ups and partial withdrawal of catheter, take it out and change to another form of analgesia.

Postoperative

Infusion regimen

Age <6m

Levobupivacaine infusion, 1.25mg/ml (0.125%) plain @ 0.1-0.2ml/kg/h ≡ 0.125-0.25mg/kg/h ≡ 125-250micrograms/kg/h

May need top ups levobupivacaine, 2.5mg/ml (0.25%) 0.1-0.3ml/kg ≡ 0.25-0.75mg/kg ≡ 250-750micrograms/kg in fractionated doses [maximum total dose (including top ups) per 4h period 1.0mg/kg]

Check block; give top up in fractionated doses; check BP,HR,RR,SpO2 every 5 minutes for 15 minutes; recheck block and pain score. Aim for differential block with preservation of motor power and good analgesia. If block is very dense with profound motor blockade, consult senior for review.

Age 6m+

Levobupivacaine infusion, 1.25mg/ml (0.125%) plain @ 0.2-0.4ml/kg/h ≡ 0.25-0.5mg/kg/h ≡ 250-500micrograms/kg/h

May need top ups levobupivacaine, 2.5mg/ml (0.25%) 0.1-0.3ml/kg ≡ 0.25-0.75mg/kg ≡ 250-750micrograms/kg in fractionated doses [maximum total dose (including top ups) per 4h period 2.0mg/kg]

Check block; give top up in fractionated doses; check BP,HR,RR,SpO2 every 5 minutes for 15 minutes; recheck block and pain score. Aim for differential block with preservation of motor power and good analgesia. If block is very dense with profound motor blockade, consult senior for review.

RESCUE ANALGESIA

If <6m use IV route for rescue analgesia and following instructions above for titration to analgesia with IV morphine.

If 6m+ place SC cannula for rescue analgesia and prescribe 0.1mg/kg (100micrograms/kg) sc morphine which can be given by ward nursing staff or ward doctor. If no sc cannula, iv morphine up to 0.1mg/kg (100micrograms/kg) can be given by ward doctor, anaesthetist or certificated nurse following instructions above for titration to analgesia with IV morphine.

ADDITIVES TO EPIDURAL SOLUTIONS

In specific cases, an additive may be mixed with levobupivacaine to prolong the analgesia from a single dose or to increase the dermatomal coverage of the block. These should only be undertaken by anaesthetists and if a trainee, discuss with your consultant and the pain team.

Fentanyl 1-2micrograms /ml of epidural infusion solution

Diamorphine 50 micrograms/kg loading dose, then solution of diamorphine, 50 microgram/ml in levobupivacaine, 1.25mg/ml (0.125%) @ 0.1ml/kg/h **max.** *[avoid if age <1y; do not increase infusion rate; top up with plain levobupivacaine; for pruritis use low dose naloxone 0.5micrograms/kg, repeated every1-2 minutes until symptoms resolve then give this total dose hourly as a continuous infusion]*

Clonidine 1 microgram/kg added to single injection blocks

Preservative free racemic ketamine (Curomed) 0.5mg/kg or S (+) ketamine 0.25-0.5mg/kg added to single injection epidural blocks [S(+)ketamine has twice the analgesic potency of racemic ketamine]

DRUGS USED IN MANAGEMENT OF EXCESSIVELY HIGH BLOCK

Use Basic Life Support measures (ABC); give oxygen; give iv fluids; call duty anaesthetist

Ephedrine 0.1-1 mg/kg IV; Atropine 10-20 micrograms/kg IV or IM

Anaesthesia, 1993, Volume 48, pages 1050–1052

An evaluation of a new self-adhesive patch preparation of amethocaine for topical anaesthesia prior to venous cannulation in children

E. DOYLE, J. FREEMAN, N. T. IM AND N. S. MORTON

Summary

A new preparation of amethocaine in the form of a self-adhesive patch, designed to provide topical cutaneous anaesthesia prior to venous cannulation, was evaluated in an open study of 189 children. The new preparation of amethocaine was in place for a mean time of 48 min (SD 3.9). Eighty percent of patients had a satisfactory degree of analgesia for venous cannulation. Nine percent of patients experienced moderate pain and 11% experienced severe pain during venous cannulation. In 26% of patients there was slight (24%) or moderate (2%) erythema at the site of application, and in 5% slight oedema was noted at the site of application. Eight percent of patients had slight itching and 1% had moderate itching at the site of application. There was a clinical impression that venous dilatation made cannulation easier than with EMLA cream. These results suggest that this convenient preparation of amethocaine is highly effective at providing adequate topical cutaneous anaesthesia with a short onset time and a low incidence of minor side effects with no evidence of systemic toxicity.

Key words

Anaesthetic techniques, regional; topical.
Veins; venipuncture.
Anaesthetics, local; amethocaine.

The provision of cutaneous topical anaesthesia prior to venepuncture or venous cannulation is clearly desirable. This is particularly so in paediatric practice when pain can make these procedures stressful for both doctor and patient. The only effective topical anaesthetic preparation currently available is a eutectic mixture of lignocaine and prilocaine (EMLA, Astra) and the efficacy of this preparation has been well demonstrated [1–6].

EMLA requires a minimum application time of 1 h under an occlusive dressing [7,8], but its anaesthetic effect is short, with a duration of 30–60 min [1,7]. There are pharmacological and experimental grounds for considering amethocaine to be a more appropriate local anaesthetic drug to use as a topical preparation than lignocaine or prilocaine [9,10].

This paper presents an open study of the efficacy, safety and side effects of a new preparation of amethocaine in the form of a self-adhesive patch applied topically prior to venous cannulation in children. This study was performed as an open evaluation rather than as a comparative trial against EMLA because it formed part of the phase II evaluation of the preparation for licensing purposes.

Methods

The study was approved by the ethics committee of the hospital. Informed written parental consent was obtained for 189 children aged between 1 and 15 years presenting for day case surgery. Exclusion criteria included lack of parental consent, weight less than 10 kg, the presence of broken skin at the site of application, known sensitivity to local anaesthetics and the use of analgesics within the preceding 24 h. All children were unpremedicated.

The weight, height, heart rate and blood pressure of each patient were recorded before drug administration. A new preparation of amethocaine in the form of a self-adhesive patch (Smith & Nephew Pharmaceuticals Ltd), incorporating a thin film of anhydrous amethocaine base 15 mg, was applied to the dorsum of one hand over a vein. The patch size was 10 cm × 6 cm and the area of drug/skin contact was 4.5 cm × 3 cm (13.5 cm^2). The specified application time was between 45 min and 1 h. Blood pressure and heart rate were recorded on removal of the amethocaine preparation and any change from the first measurement was noted.

E. Doyle, FRCA, J. Freeman, FRCA, Research Fellows, N.T. Im,* MB, BS, Registrar, N.S. Morton, FRCA, Consultant in Paediatric Anaesthesia and Intensive Care, Department of Anaesthesia, Royal Hospital for Sick Children, Yorkhill, Glasgow G3 8SJ.
*Present address: 66 Chartwell Drive, Singapore 1955.
Accepted 8 May 1993.

0003–2409/93/121050+03 $08.00/0

The patient or parent was asked about itching at the site of application and the site was inspected by the investigator for erythema and oedema. Each was graded as absent, slight or moderate. These assessments were performed by three of the investigators (E.D., J.F. and N.T.I.).

Venous cannulation was then performed using a 22- or 24-gauge cannula. The gauge of cannula used depended on the size of the vein to be cannulated and the expected ease of cannulation. An assessment of pain during cannulation was made and scored on a four-point behavioural scale previously validated in paediatric studies of injection pain due to propofol [11]: $0 =$ no pain (no grimace, crying or withdrawal of the arm); $1 =$ mild pain (grimace); $2 =$ moderate pain (grimace and cry); $3 =$ severe pain (grimace, cry and withdrawal of the arm).

A record was kept of all materials applied to the skin. Each subject was visited prior to discharge and the site of the amethocaine application inspected. The child's general practitioner was informed of his/her patient's participation in the study and asked to report any undue late problems.

Results

There were 189 applications of the test patch. Of these, 18 were invalidated because of violations of the protocol. Results from 127 males and 44 females with a mean age of 73.8 months (SD 35.3) and a mean weight of 23.4 kg (SD 10.7) were analysed.

The amethocaine patches were applied for a mean (SD) time of 48 (3.9) min. The mean (SD) time between application and cannulation was 59 (27) min. Fifty-six percent of children experienced no pain and 24% experienced mild pain on venous cannulation (Table 1). Nine percent of children experienced moderate and 11% experienced severe pain during cannulation.

At the site of amethocaine application there was mild erythema in 24% of patients and moderate erythema in 2%. Slight oedema was present in 5% of patients. Mild itching was noted in 8% of patients and moderate itching in 1%. No clinically significant haemodynamic changes were noted and there was no idiosyncratic reactions to the amethocaine.

Discussion

Our results indicate that after application times of between 45 min and 1 h this preparation of amethocaine will produce satisfactory topical cutaneous anaesthesia, that is, no reaction to cannulation or a grimace only, in 80% of children undergoing venous cannulation. The preparation may in fact have a higher success rate than this because a number of children who were scored as having severe pain

during venous cannulation (cry, grimace and withdrawal of the arm) were distressed prior to cannulation, presumably as a response to hunger or anxiety. These children may well have cried or struggled because of this rather than as a consequence of pain. This is a better result than was obtained in the early trials of EMLA [1–6]. There was a preponderance of boys in the study because paediatric day case surgery includes a high proportion of procedures such as circumcision and orchidopexy that are only performed on boys.

A short application time may be of benefit in busy wards or outpatient areas where prolonged application times disrupt the smooth running of operating lists and clinics. The known vasodilator effect of amethocaine [12,13] may produce venous dilatation and easier conditions for venepuncture than the vasoconstrictor effect that is occasionally seen with EMLA cream. Topical amethocaine appears to have a prolonged duration of action [1] persisting after the patch is removed. This may prove a useful feature in a busy setting where all the patches required for an operating session could be applied at the same time and removed at the same time. There is also the potential for prolonged wound analgesia in certain procedures such as skin grafting and the removal of minor skin blemishes.

A suitable preparation of a local anaesthetic drug for cutaneous use should provide rapid, effective and relatively long lasting anaesthesia of both the skin surface and the underlying tissues. It should also contain the minimum effective dose of drug.

The stratum corneum is the main barrier to the absorption of drugs through the skin [14]. A lipophilic local anaesthetic preparation such as the base of amethocaine should penetrate the lipid-rich barrier of the stratum corneum and block the underlying nerve fibres more readily than relatively hydrophilic preparations such as the salts of lignocaine and prilocaine which constitute EMLA cream.

There is experimental evidence to support the superiority of amethocaine over other local anaesthetics for the provision of topical cutaneous anaesthesia. When equimolar doses of amethocaine and lignocaine in the same formulation are applied to volunteers for 30 min, amethocaine provides a more significant percutaneous effect [9]. A comparison of equal doses of amethocaine and EMLA in volunteers demonstrated that the amethocaine preparation produced more rapid onset and increased duration of effect when application times of 30 and 60 min were used [1]. The greater lipophilicity and potency of amethocaine compared with lignocaine and prilocaine, and its greater affinity for neural tissue, mean that only a small amount need be present in the region of the nerve fibres to exert a phamacological action. A relatively long time after removal of the drug would be required to reduce the concentration of amethocaine present at the nerve fibres to less than that required for an anaesthetic effect. The affinity of the amethocaine molecule for the stratum corneum may result in a depot effect by which the drug remains in the skin after removal of the application and continues to diffuse through the stratum corneum into the dermis.

The use of an ester type local anaesthetic may cause concern about possible systemic toxicity especially since a highly lipophilic agent such as amethocaine base will undergo rapid systemic uptake. However, since amethocaine is an ester, it is subject to rapid metabolism by

Table 1. Pain during venous cannulation, degree of erythema, oedema and itch at site of amethocaine application.

Pain	None	Mild	Moderate	Severe	Total
	96 (56%)	41 (24%)	15 (9%)	19 (11%)	171
Erythema	Absent	Slight	Moderate		
	127 (74%)	40 (24%)	4 (2%)		171
Oedema	Absent	Slight	Moderate		
	163 (95%)	8 (5%)	0		171
Itch	Absent	Slight	Moderate		
	156 (91%)	13 (8%)	2 (1%)		171

esterases in the skin and in the blood. Thus, blood concentrations are very low [15] and dose-related systemic toxicity is unlikely. Esters are more likely than amides to produce idiosyncratic toxic effects [16] and a large series of patients will be required to determine the incidence and severity of these.

There was an incidence of slight (24%) or moderate (2%) cutaneous erythema at the site of application due to the vasodilator effect of amethocaine. This may aid identification of the application site and make venous cannulation easier. Other side effects of the application were infrequent and minor and no systemic toxicity was observed.

These results are encouraging and suggest that this preparation of amethocaine has a useful rôle in the provision of topical cutaneous anaesthesia prior to venous cannulation or venepuncture. A controlled, randomised and blind comparison with EMLA cream would be of value.

Acknowledgments

We are grateful to Smith & Nephew Pharmaceuticals Ltd for providing the amethocaine preparation used in the study. The self-adhesive patch preparation of amethocaine used in this study was developed by Smith & Nephew Research Ltd.

References

[1] McCafferty DF, Woolfson AD, Boston V. In vivo assessment of percutaneous local anaesthetic preparations. *British Journal of Anaesthesia* 1989; **62:** 17–21.

[2] Maunuksela EL, Korpela R. Double blind evaluation of a lignocaine—prilocaine cream (EMLA) in children. *British Journal of Anaesthesia* 1986; **58:** 1242–5.

[3] Ehrenstrom Reiz GME, Reiz SLA. EMLA—a eutectic mixture of local anaesthetics for topical anaesthesia. *Acta Anaesthetica Scandinavica* 1982; **26:** 596–8.

[4] Clarke S, Redfrod M. Topical anaesthetic for venepuncture. *Archives of Disease in Childhood* 1986; **61:** 1132–4.

[5] Hallen B, Uppfeldt A. Does lidocaine–prilocaine cream permit painfree insertion of IV catheters in children. *Anesthesiology* 1982; **57:** 340–2.

[6] Hopkins CS, Buckly CJ, Bush GH. Pain-free injection in infants. Use of a lignocaine–prilocaine cream to prevent pain at intravenous induction of general anaesthesia in 1–5 year old children. *Anaesthesia* 1988; **43:** 198–201.

[7] Watson K. Astra markets cream to remove pain of injections. *Pharmaceutical Journal* 1986; **236:** 262.

[8] Hallen B, Olssen GL, Uppfeldt A. Pain-free venepuncture. *Anaesthesia* 1984; **39:** 969–72.

[9] McCafferty DF, Woolfson AD, McClelland KH, Boston V. Comparative in vivo and in vitro assessment of the percutaneous absorption of local anaesthetics. *British Journal of Anaesthesia* 1988; **60:** 64–9.

[10] Covino BG. Pharmacology of local anaesthetic agents. *British Journal of Anaesthesia* 1986; **58:** 701–16.

[11] Cameron E, Johnston G, Crofts S, Morton NS. The minimum effective dose of lignocaine to abolish injection pain due to propofol in children. *Anaesthesia* 1992; **47:** 604–6.

[12] Willats DG, Reynolds F. Comparison of the vasoactivity of amide and ester local anaesthetics. *British Journal of Anaesthesia* 1985; **57:** 1006–11.

[13] Wolfson AD, McCafferty DF, McGowan KE, Boston V. Non-invasive monitoring of percutaneous local anaesthesia using Doppler velocimetry. *International Journal of Pharmaceutics* 1989; **51:** 183–7.

[14] Adriani J, Dalili H. Penetration of local anesthetics through epithelial barriers. *Anesthesia and Analgesia* 1971; **50:** 834–41.

[15] Mazumdar B, Tomlinson AA, Faulder GC. Preliminary study to assay plasma amethocaine concentrations after topical application of a new local anaesthetic cream containing amethocaine. *British Journal of Anaesthesia* 1991; **67:** 432–6.

[16] Covino BG. Toxicity of local anaesthetics. *Advances in Anaesthesia* 1986; **3:** 37–65.

Paediatric Anaesthesia 1997   7: 121–124

Plasma bupivacaine levels after fascia iliaca compartment block with and without adrenaline

E. DOYLE FRCA, N.S. MORTON FRCA AND L.R. McNICOL FRCA

Department of Anaesthesia, Royal Hospital for Sick Children, Yorkhill, Glasgow G3 8SJ, Scotland, UK

Summary

Twenty children undergoing unilateral surgery on the thigh received a fascia iliaca compartment block using $2 \, mg \cdot kg^{-1}$ of bupivacaine with (Group A) or without (Group P) adrenaline 1/200 000. Venous blood samples were taken as 5, 10, 15, 20, 25, 30, 40, 50 and 60 min after injection and assayed for concentrations of bupivacaine. In all subjects an adequate block was produced. Plasma concentrations of bupivacaine in Group P were significantly higher than those in Group A ($P<0.05$). The median maximum plasma concentration (C_{max}) was $1.1 \, \mu g \cdot ml^{-1}$ (range 0.54–$1.29 \, \mu g \cdot ml^{-1}$) in Group P and $0.35 \, \mu g \cdot ml^{-1}$ (range 0.17–$0.96 \, \mu g \cdot ml^{-1}$) in Group A. The median time taken to attain C_{max} (T_{max}) was 20 min (range 10–25 min) in Group P and 45 min (range 5–50 min) in Group A. The median time to first analgesia was 9.75 h (range 3–15 h) in Group P and 10.5 h (range 2.5–21 h) in Group A. The study confirmed the efficacy of the fascia iliaca compartment block in children and showed that when performed with $2 \, mg \cdot kg^{-1}$ of bupivacaine it is associated with plasma concentrations of bupivacaine well within acceptable limits. The addition of adrenaline 1/200 000 to the local anaesthetic solution reduces the maximum plasma concentration reached.

Keywords: paediatric; analgesia; fascia iliaca block; bupivacaine; adrenaline

Introduction

The fascia iliaca compartment block has been described as an alternative to femoral nerve block and 'three-in-one' block for the provision of unilateral analgesia in the lower limbs (1). The technique involves injection of local anaesthetic solution into the fascia iliaca compartment which is a potential space between the iliacus muscle and the fascia iliaca

which covers it. This space is limited anteriorly by the fascia iliaca, posteriorly by the iliacus muscle, medially by the vertebral column and upper sacrum and laterally by the inner surface of the iliac crest. Distally the fascia iliaca blends with the fascia covering sartorius and is covered by fascia lata below the inguinal ligament and so the fascia iliaca compartment extends to the lateral part of the upper thigh. The femoral, obturator and lateral cutaneous nerves traverse the fascia iliaca compartment and can be blocked by local anaesthetic solution deposited in this compartment in the thigh if a sufficient volume is injected and upward migration is encouraged by

Correspondence to: Dr E. Doyle, Department of Anaesthesia, Royal Hospital for Sick Children, Sciennes Road, Edinburgh EH9 1LF, Scotland, UK.

the application distal pressure. The fascia iliaca compartment block does not require the use of a nerve stimulator or the production of parathesiae and is performed away from blood vessels and nerves so that the chances of inadvertent nerve injury or intravascular injection of local anaesthetic are remote. The technique has been shown to have a significantly higher success rate (95%) than the 'three-in-one' block in children (20%) (1).

The technique requires a significant dose of local anaesthetic solution near the maximum of $2.5 \, mg \cdot kg^{-1}$ when bupivacaine is used and there are no data on the plasma levels reached when these doses are used for the fascia iliaca compartment block. This study was carried out to determine the plasma concentrations reached when the fascia iliaca compartment block is performed in children with $2 \, mg \cdot kg^{-1}$ of 0.25% bupivacaine with and without adrenaline.

Methods

The study was approved by the hospital ethics committee and written informed parental consent was obtained for each child recruited in to the study. Twenty children aged from 1 to 14 years undergoing unilateral removal of a femoral plate were recruited. Subjects were premedicated with EMLA cream one hour preoperatively and anaesthesia was induced with propofol $3-4 \, mg \cdot kg^{-1}$. A laryngeal mask airway was inserted and anaesthesia maintained with isoflurane 0.5–2% with 70% nitrous oxide in oxygen. A second intravenous cannula was then sited for blood sampling.

A fascia iliaca compartment block was performed at a point 1–2 cm perpendicularly below the junction of the lateral one third and medial two thirds of the inguinal ligament. A 22 G short bevelled regional block needle was connected to a syringe of local anaesthetic solution by a length of plastic tubing and inserted perpendicular to the skin and advanced slowly until a distinct double pop was felt as it pierced first the fascia lata and then the fascia iliaca. After a negative aspiration test the local anaesthetic solution was injected while firm pressure was exerted distal to the injection site. The dose used was $2 \, mg \cdot kg^{-1}$ (0.8 ml·kg^{-1}) of 0.25% bupivacaine. Patients were randomly allocated to receive either plain bupivacaine (Group P) or commercially

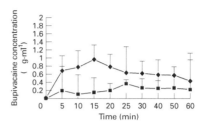

Figure 1
Plasma concentrations (median range) of bupivacaine in Groups P and A. ◆ Plain; ■ Adrenaline.

available (Astra Pharmaceuticals) bupivacaine + 1/200 000 adrenaline (Group A).

Following injection, venous blood samples (1 ml) were taken at 5, 10, 15, 20, 25, 30, 40, 50 and 60 min. These were taken after removal of 5 ml of 'dead space' blood and immediately placed in crushed ice. Samples were centrifuged at 4°C for 15 min and the plasma removed and stored at -20°C until analysis. Plasma samples were made alkaline by the addition of 0.5 ml of 1 M NaOH and extracted with 6 ml of diethyl ether. The ethereal layer was transferred to a tapered glass tube containing 1 ml 1 M HCl. The samples and standards were roller mixed for 20 min and the ether layer removed and discarded. The remaining solution was make alkaline by the addition of 1 ml 4 M NaOH and finally extracted in 75 μl of chloroform. Aliquots of 1 μl were then injected directly onto the high performance liquid chromatography column. Peak height ratios for the drug and internal standard were used to construct a standard graph of concentration versus peak height ratio. An external quality control was run in conjunction with each batch of analyses.

When patients had recovered from anaesthesia the presence of an adequate block was tested by skin pinching in the appropriate areas. The duration of the block was taken as the time to administration of first postoperative analgesia as determined by a request for analgesia from parent or child.

Statistical analysis was performed with Student's t-test for parametric data (age and weight) and the Mann-Whitney U-test for bupivacaine concentrations.

Results

The samples from one patient were lost and this subject was excluded from the results of the study.

© 1997 Blackwell Science Ltd, *Paediatric Anaesthesia*, **7**, 121–124

Table 1
Demographic and operative data on patients in Groups P and A

	Group P	Group A
Age/yrs Mean (SD)	7.7 (4.2)	7.6 (4.1)
Weight/kg Mean (SD)	26.8 (10.2)	30 (14.8)
M:F	4:5	4:6
L:R	5:4	4:6

The two groups were comparable in terms of demographic characteristics and operative procedures (Table 1).

All subjects in both groups were pain free on recovery from anaesthesia and were demonstrated to have an appropriate area of sensory blockade at this time.

Plasma concentrations of bupivacaine were compared and are illustrated in Figure 1.

Plasma concentrations of bupivacaine in Group P were significantly higher than those in Group A at all times ($P<0.05$). The median maximum plasma concentration (C_{max}) was $1.1\,\mu g \cdot ml^{-1}$ (range $0.54-1.29\,\mu g \cdot ml^{-1}$) in Group P and $0.35\,\mu g \cdot ml^{-1}$ (range $0.17-0.96\,\mu g \cdot ml^{-1}$) in Group A. The median time taken to attain (C_{max}) (T_{max}) was 20 min (range 10–25 min) in Group P and 45 min (range 5–50 min) in Group A.

One subject in Group P did not ask for further analgesia. The median time to first analgesia in the remaining subjects was 9.75 h (range 3–15 h) in Group P and 10.5 h (range 2.5–21 h) in Group A. It was felt that the Groups were too small for statistical comparisons of the duration of analgesia to be useful.

Discussion

This study has confirmed the efficacy of the fascia iliaca compartment block when performed in children to provide analgesia for unilateral surgery on the leg. This is the first study to measure plasma levels of bupivacaine after this technique and the plasma levels of bupivacaine after the use of $2\,mg \cdot kg^{-1}$ are low and well below the level of $4\,\mu g \cdot ml^{-1}$ at which toxicity is likely to occur (2,3). These values are similar to those seen after caudal epidural analgesia in children with $2\,mg \cdot kg^{-1}$ (4), $3\,mg \cdot kg^{-1}$ (5), $3.1\,mg \cdot kg^{-1}$ (6) and $3.7\,mg \cdot kg^{-1}$ (7) of

bupivacaine. The median times taken to reach these levels are similar to those seen in studies of caudal epidural analgesia in children where the times taken range from 15 to 45 min (4,5,7–9) compared with less than 10 min after intercostal injection of bupivacaine in infants (9,10). These figures suggest that the fascia iliaca compartment is a relatively avascular space compared with the intercostal space and that the absorption of local anaesthetics from it is relatively slow and may be further reduced by the use of adrenaline containing solutions.

No attempt was made to follow the elimination curve of bupivacaine in this study because the elimination characteristics of bupivacaine in healthy children are well described (9,11).

The addition of adrenaline to bupivacaine did not appear to prolong the duration of the fascia iliaca compartment blocks in this study.

In summary, this study has confirmed the efficacy of the fascia iliaca compartment block in children and shown that when performed with $2\,mg \cdot kg^{-1}$ of bupivacaine is associated with plasma concentrations of bupivacaine well within acceptable limits. The addition of adrenaline 1/200 000 to the local anaesthetic solution reduces the maximum plasma concentration reached but does not appear to prolong the duration of the block.

Acknowledgement

We are grateful to Iain McDonald and Mark Drottar of the Department of Anaesthesia, University of Glasgow for performing the bupivacaine assays in this study.

References

1 Dalens B, Vanneuville G, Tanguy A. Comparison of the fascia iliaca compartment block with the 3-in-1 block in children. *Anesth Analg* 1989; **69**: 705–713.
2 Mather LE, Long GJ, Thomas J. The intravenous toxicity and clearance of bupivacaine in man. *Clin Pharmacol Therapeut* 1971; **12**: 935–943.
3 Moore DC, Balfour RI, Fitzgibbons D. Convulsive arterial plasma levels of bupivacaine and the response to diazepam therapy. *Anesthesiology* 1979; **50**: 454–456.
4 Eyres RL, Kidd J, Oppenheim R *et al.* Local anaesthetic plasma levels in children. *Anaesth Intens Care* 1978; **6**: 243–247.
5 Eyres RL, Bishop W, Oppenheim RC *et al.* Plasma bupivacaine concentrations in children during caudal epidural analgesia. *Anaesth Intens Care* 1983; **11**: 20–22.

6 Armitage EN. Caudal block in children. *Anaesthesia* 1979; **34**: 396.

7 Takasaki M. Blood concentrations of lidocaine, mepivacaine and bupivacaine during caudal analgesia in children. *Acta Anesthes Scand* 1984; **28**: 211–214.

8 Stow PJ, Scott A, Phillips A. Plasma bupivacaine concentrations during caudal analgesia and ilioinguinal-hypogastric nerve block in children. *Anaesthesia* 1988; **43**: 650–653.

9 Rothstein P, Arthur FR, Feldman HS *et al.* Bupivacaine for intercostal nerve blocks in children: blood concentrations and pharmacokinetics. *Anesth Analg* 1986; **65**: 625–632.

10 Bricker SRW, Telford RJ, Booker PD. Pharmacokinetics of bupivacaine following intraoperative intercostal nerve block in neonates and in infants aged less than 6 months. *Anesthesiology* 1989; **70**: 942–947.

11 Mazoit JX, Denson DD, Samii K. Pharmacokinetics of bupivacaine following caudal analgesia in infants. *Anesthesiology* 1986; **68**: 387–391.

Accepted 7 June 1996

Paediatric Anaesthesia 1998   8: 467–471

Tracheal intubation without neuromuscular blockade in children: a comparison of propofol combined either with alfentanil or remifentanil

D.N. ROBINSON MBChB, FRCA, BSc, K. O'BRIEN MBChB, FFARCSI,
R. KUMAR MBBS, FRCA AND N.S. MORTON MBChB, FRCA, FRCPCH
Department of Anaesthesia, Royal Hospital for Sick Children, Yorkhill, Glasgow G3 8SJ, Scotland, UK

Summary

Forty healthy children, aged between two and 12 years of age undergoing elective surgery where the anaesthetic technique involved tracheal intubation followed by spontaneous ventilation were studied. Induction of anaesthesia was with either alfentanil 15 µg·kg^{-1} or remifentanil 1 µg·kg^{-1} followed by propofol 4 mg·kg^{-1} to which lignocaine 0.2 mg·kg^{-1} had been added. Intubating conditions were graded on a four point scale for ease of laryngoscopy, vocal cord position, degree of coughing, jaw relaxation and limb movement. All children were successfully intubated at the first attempt. There were no significant differences in the assessments of intubating conditions between the two groups. Arterial blood pressure and heart changes were similar in the two groups with both alfentanil and remifentanil attenuating the haemodynamic response to tracheal intubation. The time taken to resumption of spontaneous ventilation was similar in both groups.

Keywords: anaesthetics, intravenous: propofol; analgesics, opioid: alfentanil; remifentanil; intubation: tracheal

Introduction

The use of suxamethonium to facilitate tracheal intubation may give rise to adverse effects. This has led to a decline in its role in anaesthesia for elective paediatric surgery. The combined use of propofol and alfentanil to facilitate elective tracheal intubation is well established in both adult (1–5) and paediatric practice (6–9). Remifentanil is a recently introduced potent opioid that has a short blood brain

equilibration time and is rapidly hydrolysed by nonspecific esterases in the blood resulting in a fast offset of action. These pharmacological properties suggest that remifentanil may be a suitable opioid to use, in combination with propofol, to facilitate tracheal intubation when a rapid return to spontaneous ventilation is required. This study was designed to compare intubating conditions, haemodynamic response and the time taken to resumption of spontaneous ventilation following the use of either alfentanil or remifentanil combined with propofol to facilitate tracheal intubation in children.

Correspondence to: N.S. Morton, Department of Anaesthesia, Royal Hospital for Sick Children, Yorkhill, Glasgow G3 8SJ, Scotland, UK.

Patients and methods

Local ethics committee approval was obtained to study 40 children, aged 2–12 years of age, who would require tracheal intubation as part of their anaesthetic technique and in whom spontaneous ventilation was planned during surgery. All patients were ASA I or II. Patients were excluded if history or examination suggested difficulty in intubation. Informed written consent was obtained from a parent of all patients studied. Premedication consisted of trimeprazine 2 mg·kg⁻¹, given one to two h prior to surgery, and the application of EMLA cream to the dorsum of each hand at the same time. On arrival in the anaesthetic room, baseline noninvasive measurements of heart rate, arterial blood pressure and pulse oximeter oxygen saturation (SpO_2) were made. A 22 G cannula was sited on the dorsum of a hand. Patients were then randomly assigned to one of two groups: in Group 1, anaesthesia was induced with alfentanil 15 μg·kg⁻¹ given over 30 s, followed by propofol 4 mg·kg⁻¹ given over 15 s. Lignocaine 0.2 mg·kg⁻¹ was mixed with the propofol to prevent pain on injection. In Group 2, anaesthesia was induced with remifentanil 1 μg·kg⁻¹ given over 30 s, followed by propofol as for Group 1. In both groups, following completion of the propofol injection, the lungs were ventilated with 67% nitrous oxide in oxygen and, at 45 s following completion of the propofol injection, tracheal intubation was attempted by an experienced paediatric anaesthetist blinded to the patient's randomization group. Following tracheal intubation, isoflurane 1% inspired was added to the fresh gas and ventilation was supported until spontaneous breathing resumed. At this point the study was complete. Recordings of heart rate, arterial blood pressure and SpO_2 were made immediately following induction of anaesthesia and at one and three min following tracheal intubation. The quality of intubating conditions obtained was graded using the scoring system of Helbo-Hansen (10), as modified by Steyn (8). Ease of laryngoscopy, vocal cord position, degree of coughing, jaw relaxation and limb movement were scored on a four-point scale (Table 1). Overall intubating conditions were defined as, 'near ideal', when at worse there was a single score of two in any category, and as, 'suboptimal', when at best there was a single score of three in any category.

Power calculations showed that, in order to detect a difference of two min in the mean time to resumption of spontaneous ventilation at a two tailed significance of 5% with 90% power, 15 patients would be required in each group. Similarly, to detect a halving in the proportion of patients who were considered to have 'near ideal' intubating conditions at a two tailed significance of 5% with 90% power, would require 22 patients in each group. Twenty patients in each group were studied.

The results were analysed using SPSS statistical software. Interval data were examined for normality using normal plots and Lilliefors testing. Groups were then compared using two sample t-testing or Mann-Whitney U-testing as appropriate. For nominal data, groups were compared using the chi-square test or Fisher's exact test as appropriate. Results were considered significant when $P<0.05$.

Results

A total of 40 children was studied, divided equally between the alfentanil and remifentanil groups. The two groups were comparable in age, weight and gender distribution (Table 2). In all patients, intubation was successful at the first attempt. The scores obtained for each assessment category are shown in Table 3. 'Near ideal', overall intubating conditions were obtained in 17/20 and 16/20 patients in the alfentanil and remifentanil groups respectively. Overall, 'suboptimal', intubating conditions were obtained in 2/20 and 4/20 patients in the alfentanil and remifentanil groups respectively. There were no significant differences between the groups for individual assessment categories nor for the overall assessments of intubating conditions. Haemodynamic changes are summarized in Figure 1 and Figure 2. There were no significant differences between the two groups. Remifentanil produced a greater fall in mean arterial pressure following induction of anaesthesia but this did not reach statistical significance. There were no episodes of clinically significant bradycardia in any patients. Episodes of oxygen desaturation (SpO_2 <95%) occurred in 3/20 patients in the alfentanil group and in 4/20 patients in the remifentanil group. In all cases, these episodes were related to upper airway obstruction in patients having adenotonsillectomy and were rapidly resolved by the use of a Guedel

Table 1
Scoring system used for intubating conditions

	Score			
	1	2	3	4
Laryngoscopy	Easy	Fair	Difficult	Impossible
Vocal cords	Open	Moving	Closing	Closed
Coughing	None	Slight	Moderate	Severe
Jaw relaxation	Complete	Slight	Stiff	Rigid
Limb movement	None	Slight	Moderate	Severe

Table 2
Patient demographics (median [range] or number)

n	Alfentanil group 20	Remifentanil group 20	P
Age (months)	80 [31–142]	64 [29–123]	NS
Weight (kg)	21 [14–42]	20 [11–42]	NS
Gender (m/f)	7/13	7/13	

Table 3
Number of patients in each group given each score by category. (No patient received a score of four in any category.)

	Score = 1	Score = 2	Score = 3
Alfentanil group			
Laryngoscopy	20	–	–
Vocal cords	20	–	–
Coughing	16	2	2
Jaw relaxation	20	–	–
Limb movement	15	5	–
Remifentanil group			
Laryngoscopy	20	–	–
Vocal cords	19	1	–
Coughing	13	3	4
Jaw relaxation	20	–	–
Limb movement	14	6	–

airway. No patient exhibited chest wall rigidity which interfered with ventilation of the lungs. The median time to resumption of spontaneous ventilation in the alfentanil group was 365 s (range 100–588 s) and, in the remifentanil group, 347 s (range 146–492 s).

Discussion

The use of remifentanil has been reported in paediatric practice (11,12), though experience is still limited. Because of its very short elimination half-time, remifentanil is normally administered as a

© 1998 Blackwell Science Ltd, *Paediatric Anaesthesia*, **8**, 467–471

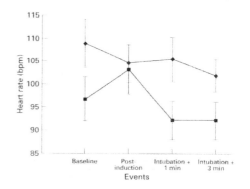

Figure 1
Changes in heart rate. Values are mean (SEM) for the alfentanil group (■) and the remifentanil group (◆).

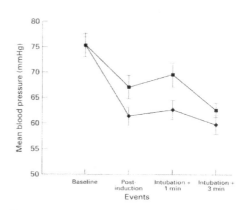

Figure 2
Changes in mean arterial pressure. Values are mean (SEM) for the alfentanil group (■) and the remifentanil group (◆).

continuous infusion during surgery. In this study, we restricted our use of remifentanil to a single bolus to assess its effect compared to alfentanil, when combined with propofol in facilitating intubation. Previous studies, in children, using propofol alone, found intubating conditions to be inadequate (6,8). Therefore, a control group using propofol without opioid was not used.

All opioids have the potential to produce dose dependent falls in blood pressure and heart rate. Previous studies using higher doses of alfentanil (greater than 30 μg·kg⁻¹) to facilitate intubation have shown that hypotension and bradycardia may occur (13,14). In our study, following induction of anaesthesia patients in the remifentanil group showed a larger fall in mean arterial pressure, but this did not reach statistical significance. A previous study (12) included a comparison of remifentanil and alfentanil in paediatric patients undergoing daycase strabismus surgery. The bolus dose of alfentanil used was 100 μg·kg⁻¹, and for remifentanil 1 μg·kg⁻¹. Hypotension was not reported following induction of anaesthesia, but of the 19 patients who received the above bolus of alfentanil, followed by an infusion at 2.5 μg·kg⁻¹·min⁻¹, four required naloxone after the termination of anaesthesia, and a further four patients had postoperative hypoxaemia, attributed to opioid induced respiratory depression. For our study, we aimed to give equivalent doses of opioid. Using published pharmacodynamic data, that were available for adults, we took remifentanil as being 15 times as potent as alfentanil (15). Subsequently, remifentanil has been reported as being between 7.7 to 30 times as potent as alfentanil (16–18).

We chose to administer the opioid while the patients were awake, and intubation was timed to take place 75 s following the start of induction. The $t_{1/2}$ke0 (the half-time for equilibration between plasma and the effect compartment) of remifentanil for analgesia has been calculated as 1.3 min (19). Therefore, the peak effect should have occurred at the time of laryngoscopy. Chest wall rigidity has been reported following the administration of remifentanil to awake adults (20). It is interesting that we did not encounter this with our paediatric patients. Chest wall rigidity is associated with rapid administration of opioid, and in our study the administration of remifentanil and alfentanil over 30 s may have conferred some protection.

The time to resumption of spontaneous ventilation was similar in both groups. Although remifentanil has a very short elimination half-life of 9.5 min, compared to 58 min for alfentanil (19), recovery of spontaneous ventilation following a single bolus dose of drug, as was used in this study, is likely to be due to drug redistribution—the $t_{1/2}$, for remifentanil and alfentanil are similar at 0.83 and 0.79 min respectively (15).

Lignocaine has been shown to improve intubating conditions in both adult and paediatric studies, largely by a reduction in the incidence and severity of coughing. The efficacy of lignocaine to suppress the cough reflex increases in a dose-dependent manner and correlates well with plasma concentrations (21,22). In this study, we used lignocaine 0.2 mg·kg⁻¹ which has been shown to be the minimum effective dose required to prevent injection pain due to propofol (23). It is unlikely that, at this dose, intubating conditions were significantly affected. Conversely, the use of a larger dose of lignocaine might be effective in improving intubation conditions, with particular regard to cough.

Conclusions

In summary, we have shown that in children remifentanil 1 μg·kg⁻¹, followed by propofol 4 mg·kg⁻¹, provides intubating conditions which are comparable to those provided by alfentanil 15 μg·kg⁻¹, followed by the same dose of propofol. Remifentanil does not appear to offer any advantage when compared to alfentanil for routine use, but when the use of an intraoperative infusion of remifentanil is planned, it may conveniently be used to facilitate intubation at induction of anaesthesia.

References

1 Scheller MS, Zornow MH, Saidman LJ. Tracheal intubation without the use of muscle relaxants: a technique using propofol and varying doses of alfentanil. *Anesth Analg* 1992; 75: 788–793.
2 Beck GN, Masterson GR, Richards J *et al.* Comparison of intubation following propofol and alfentanil with intubation following thiopentone and suxamethonium. *Anaesthesia* 1993; 48: 876–880.
3 Alcock R, Peachey T, Lynch M *et al.* Comparison of alfentanil with suxamethonium in facilitating nasotracheal intubation in day-case anaesthesia. *Br J Anaesth* 1993; 70: 34–37.
4 Coghlan SFE, McDonald PF, Csepregi G. Use of alfentanil with propofol for nasotracheal intubation without neuromuscular block. *Br J Anaesth* 1993; 70: 89–91.

5 Davidson JAH, Gillespie JA. Tracheal intubation after induction of anaesthesia with propofol, alfentanil and i.v. lignocaine. *Br J Anaesth* 1993; **70**: 163–166.

6 Rodney GE, Reichert CC, O'Regan DN *et al.* Propofol or propofol/alfentanil compared to thiopentone/succinylcholine for intubation of healthy children. *Can J Anaesth* 1992; **39**: A129.

7 Hiller A, Klemola UM, Saarnivaara L. Tracheal intubation after induction of anaesthesia with propofol, alfentanil and lidocaine without neuromuscular block in children. *Acta Anaesthesiol Scand* 1993; **37**: 725–729.

8 Steyn MP, Quinn AM, Gillespie JA *et al.* Tracheal intubation without neuromuscular block in children. *Br J Anaesth* 1994; **72**: 403–406.

9 McConaghy P, Bunting HE. Assessment of intubating conditions in children after induction with propofol and varying doses of alfentanil. *Br J Anaesth* 1994; **73**: 596–599.

10 Helbo-Hansen S, Ravlo O, Trap-Anderson S. The influence of alfentanil in the intubating conditions after priming with vecuronium. *Acta Anaesthesiol Scand* 1988; **32**: 41–44.

11 Davis PJ, Ross A, Stiller RL *et al.* Pharmacokinetics of remifentanil in anesthetized children aged 2–12 years of age. *Anesth Analg* 1995; **80**: S93.

12 Davis PJ, Lerman J, Suresh S *et al.* A randomized multicentre study of remifentanil compared with alfentanil, isoflurane, or propofol in anesthetized pediatric patients undergoing elective strabismus surgery. *Anesth Analg* 1997; **84**: 982–989.

13 Martineau RJ, Tousignant CP, Miller DR *et al.* Alfentanil controls the haemodynamic response during rapid-sequence induction of anaesthesia. *Can J Anaesth* 1990; **37**: 755–761.

14 Lindgren L, Rautiainen P, Klemola UM *et al.* Haemodynamic responses and prolongation of QT interval of ECG after suxamethonium-facilitated intubation during anaesthetic induction of children: a dose related attenuation by alfentanil. *Acta Anaesthesiol Scand* 1991; **35**: 355–358.

15 Egan TD, Minto C, Lemmens HMJ *et al.* Remifentanil versus alfentanil: comparative pharmacodynamics. *Anesthesiology* 1994; **81**: A374.

16 Egan TD, Minto CF, Hermann DJ *et al.* Remifentanil versus alfentanil: comparative pharmacokinetics in healthy adult male volunteers. *Anesthesiology* 1996; **84**: 821–833.

17 Jhaveri R, Joshi P, Batenhorst R *et al.* Dose comparison of remifentanil and alfentanil for loss of consciousness. *Anesthesiology* 1997; **87**: 253–259.

18 Hoke JF, Cunningham F, James MK *et al.* Comparative pharmacokinetics and pharmacodynamics of remifentanil, its principle metabolite (GR90291) and alfentanil in dogs. *J Pharmacol Exp Ther* 1997; **281**: 226–232.

19 Glass PS, Hardman D, Kamiyama Y *et al.* Preliminary pharmacokinetics and pharmacodynamics of an ultra-short-acting opioid: remifentanil (GI87084B). *Anesth Analg* 1993; **77**: 1031–1040.

20 Schuttler J, Albrecht S, Breivik H. A comparison of remifentanil and alfentanil in patients undergoing major abdominal surgery. *Anaesthesia* 1997; **52**: 307–317.

21 Yukioka H, Yoshimoto N, Nishimura K *et al.* Intravenous lidocaine as a suppressant of coughing during tracheal intubation. *Anesth Analg* 1985; **64**: 1189–1192.

22 Mulholland D, Carlisle RJT. Intubation with propofol augmented with intravenous lignocaine. *Anaesthesia* 1991; **46**: 312–313.

23 Cameron E, Johnston G, Crofts S *et al.* The minimum effective dose of lignocaine to abolish injection pain due to propofol in children. *Anaesthesia* 1992; **47**: 604–606.

Accepted 13 February 1998

Anaesthesia, 1992, Volume 47, pages 604–606

Forum

The minimum effective dose of lignocaine to prevent injection pain due to propofol in children

E. Cameron, MA, MRCP, FRCAnaes, Registrar, G. Johnston, MB, ChB, FRCAnaes, Senior Registrar, S. Crofts, MB, ChB, FRCAnaes, Registrar, N.S. Morton, MB, ChB, FFARCS, Consultant, Department of Anaesthesia, Royal Hospital for Sick Children, Glasgow G3 8SJ.

Summary

In a single-blind study of 100 children aged 1 to 10 years, the minimum effective dose of lignocaine required to prevent injection pain due to propofol was 0.2 mg.kg⁻¹ when veins on the dorsum of the hand were used. This is more than twice the adult value. We concluded that injection pain should not limit the use of propofol in children if an adequate amount of lignocaine is mixed immediately prior to injection.

Key words

Anaesthetics, intravenous; propofol.
Anaesthetics local; lignocaine.
Complications; pain

Injection pain is the commonest problem encountered when propofol is administered, occurring in up to 73% of adults [1], and 85% of children [2]. One successful strategy for pain prevention is the addition of lignocaine to propofol immediately before injection [3, 4]. In a group of 50 unpremedicated children, lignocaine (1 mg.kg⁻¹) mixed with propofol (3 mg.kg⁻¹) resulted in abolition of injection pain [5]. However, this dose of lignocaine was chosen empirically and the aim of the present study was to determine the minimum effective dose of lignocaine.

Methods

The study was approved by the hospital Ethics Committee and was carried out under the automatic exemption conditions of the Medicines Act 1965 (revised 1985) [6]. Informed consent was obtained from the parents of 100 children, 50 aged 1 to < 5 years and 50 aged 5 to < 10 years. Children with known sensitivity to local anaesthetics, egg protein, soya bean emulsion or a significant history of atopy were specifically not studied. No sedative or anticholinergic premedication was used but all children had EMLA cream applied to the dorsum of each hand at least 1 h before venous cannulation (22 gauge Venflon, Vygon UK).

Propofol 3 mg.kg⁻¹ was drawn up into a syringe and lignocaine was mixed immediately before injection according to the following scheme: the first child in each age group received lignocaine 1 mg.kg⁻¹. If no pain on injection was observed then the next child received a dose of lignocaine reduced by 0.1 mg.kg⁻¹. This sequence was followed until pain was observed when the next patient received 0.1 mg.kg⁻¹ increased dose of lignocaine.

Injection pain was assessed by an observer who was unaware of the lignocaine dose used. A four point beha-

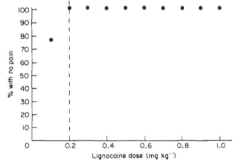

Fig. 1. Percentage of children aged 1 to 10 years where no pain was observed at each lignocaine dose level. No child who received 0.2 mg.kg⁻¹ or more experienced pain. 22.5% of children who received 0.1 mg.kg⁻¹ experienced pain.

vioural rating scale was used (no pain = 0; mild pain (grimace) = 1; moderate pain (grimace + cry) = 2; severe pain (cry + withdraw limb) = 3).

Results

One hundred children were studied. Their median age was 5.5 years (range 1.08–9.83) and their median weight was 22.7 kg (range 9.7–35.7). The proportion of children in whom no injection pain occurred is detailed for each dose level of lignocaine in Figure 1. No child was assessed as having injection pain who received 0.2 mg.kg⁻¹ or more of

Correspondence should be addressed to Dr N. S. Morton, please.
Accepted 12 February 1992.

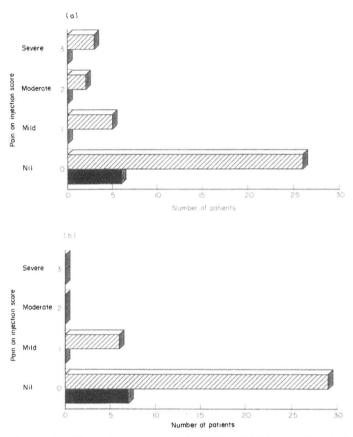

Fig. 2(a). Pain on injection scores for children aged 1 to < 5 years receiving 0.1 (▨) and 0.2 (■) mg.kg⁻¹ lignocaine (0 = no pain; 1 = mild pain; 2 = moderate pain; 3 = severe pain). (b) Pain on injection scores for children aged 5 to 10 years receiving 0.1 (▨) and 0.2 (■) mg.kg⁻¹ lignocaine (0 = no pain; 1 = mild pain; 2 = moderate pain; 3 = severe pain). If pain on injection was experienced, it tended to be more severe in younger children, aged 1 to < 5 years.

lignocaine. 22.5% of children who had received 0.1 mg.kg⁻¹ lignocaine were assessed as having injection pain. Pain was assessed as being moderate or severe in five patients in the 1 to < 5 year age group (Figs 2(a) and (b)).

Discussion

One method of preventing injection pain due to propofol in adults, is to use a large antecubital vein [4]. In children, this results in injection pain in 6.6% [7] to 24% [8]. However, the antecubital fossa carries the risk of arterial or neural damage and in children the availability of EMLA cream has made painless cannulation of veins on the dorsum of the hand the preferred choice of most anaesthetists.

This study confirmed the efficacy of added lignocaine in preventing injection pain due to propofol. However, an adequate dose must be used in children where 22.5% of 1 to 10 year olds experienced pain despite the addition of 0.1 mg.kg⁻¹ lignocaine to 3 mg.kg⁻¹ propofol. In younger children aged 1 to 5 years, injection pain tends to be more severe. In adults, the minimum effective dose of lignocaine

to prevent injection pain is 0.08 mg.kg⁻¹ (0.025%) [9], whereas our study indicates that for children aged 1 to 10 years, 0.2 mg.kg⁻¹ is required. Thus, children's veins would appear to be twice as susceptible to this adverse effect of propofol.

Previous studies in children have used an adaptation of the recommended adult regimen of 10 mg lignocaine per 200 mg propofol [10, 11]. At an induction dose of 3 mg.kg⁻¹ this produces a lignocaine dose of 0.15 mg.kg⁻¹. However, these studies found an incidence of injection pain of 29% and 60% respectively. Efficacy of added lignocaine is known to decline after 30 min [12] and it is possible that mixing immediately before administration in the present study was responsible for the efficacy of 0.2 mg.kg⁻¹. Any delay between mixing lignocaine with propofol and administration may result in a critical reduction in the concentration of lignocaine in the nonlipid phase of the emulsion, i.e. in the amount available to block afferent nerve fibres in the vein wall [13].

We conclude that the minimum effective dose of lignocaine required to prevent injection pain due to propofol

3 mg.kg^{-1} in children is 0.2 mg.kg^{-1}. Injection pain is not a problem in children who receive propofol if an adequate amount of lignocaine is mixed with the propofol immediately before administration.

References

[1] JOHNSON RA, HARPER NJN, CHADWICK S, VOHRA A. Pain on injection of propofol: methods of alleviation. *Anaesthesia* 1990; **45**: 439–42.

[2] VALTONEN M, IISALO E, KANTO J, TIKKANEN J. Propofol as an induction agent in children: pain on injection and pharmacokinetics. *Acta Anaesthesiologica Scandinavica* 1989; **33**: 152–5.

[3] REDFERN N, STAFFORD MA, HULL CJ. Incremental propofol for short procedures. *British Journal of Anaesthesia* 1985; **57**: 1178–82.

[4] SCOTT RPF, SAUNDERS DA, NORMAN J. Propofol: clinical strategies for preventing the pain on injection. *Anaesthesia* 1988; **43**: 492–4.

[5] MORTON NS. Abolition of injection pain due to propofol in children. *Anaesthesia* 1990; **45**: 70.

[6] Department of Health and Social Security. Medicines Act Leaflet MAL30. DHSS Medicines Division 1985: London.

[7] HANNALLAH RS, BAKER SB, CASEY W, McGILL WA, BROADMAN LM, NORDEN JM. Propofol: effective dose and induction characteristics in unpremedicated children. *Anesthesiology* 1991; **74**: 217–20.

[8] PURCELL-JONES G, YATES A, BAKER JR, JAMES IG. Comparison of the induction characteristics of thiopentone and propofol in children. *British Journal of Anaesthesia* 1987; **59**: 1431–6.

[9] STAFFORD MA, HULL CJ, WAGSTAFF A. Effect of lignocaine on pain during injection of propofol. *British Journal of Anaesthesia* 1991; **66**: 406–7P.

[10] PATEL DK, KEELING PA, NEWMAN GB, RADFORD P. Induction dose of propofol in children. *Anaesthesia* 1988; **43**: 949–52.

[11] MORTON NS, WEE M, CHRISTIE G, GRAY IG, GRANT IS. Propofol for induction of anaesthesia in children. A comparison with thiopentone and halothane inhalational induction. *Anaesthesia* 1988; **43**: 350–5.

[12] GLEN JB. The animal pharmacology of ICI 35868: a new i.v. anaesthetic agent. *British Journal of Anaesthesia* 1980; **52**: 230P.

[13] KLEMENT W, ARNDT JO. Pain on i.v. injection of some anaesthetic agents is evoked by the unphysiological osmolality or pH of their formulations. *British Journal of Anaesthesia* 1991; **66**: 189–95.

Journal of Pharmaceutical & Biomedical Analysis, Vol. 13, No. 1, pp. 27–32, 1995
Elsevier Science Ltd
Printed in Great Britain
0731-7085/95 $9.50 + 0.00

Pergamon

0731-7085(94)00121-9

Analysis of unconjugated morphine, codeine, normorphine and morphine as glucuronides in small volumes of plasma from children

D.G. WATSON,*† Q. SU,† J.M. MIDGLEY,† E. DOYLE‡ and N.S. MORTON‡

† Department of Pharmaceutical Sciences, University of Strathclyde, Glasgow G1 1XW, UK
‡ Department of Anaesthesia, Royal Hospital for Sick Children, Yorkhill, Glasgow G3 8SJ, UK

Abstract: A sensitive method for the analysis of unconjugated morphine, codeine, normorphine and total morphine after hydrolysis of glucuronide conjugates is described. The method was applicable to 50-μl volumes of plasma. The analytes were converted to heptafluorobutyryl (HFB) derivatives before analysis by gas chromatography–negative ion chemical ionization mass spectrometry. Morphine and codeine were quantified against their [$^2H_3$]-isotopomers. Linearity, precision and accuracy were quite acceptable (in the 10^{-10}–10^{-9} g range), and the absolute limits of detection were <1 pg.

Keywords: GC–MS; morphine; morphine glucuronides; codeine; normorphine.

Introduction

Post-operative relief of pain in children has been carried out using opioids in a continuous infusion for a number of years [1]. The subcutaneous route for delivery of the drug has been used for many years in the terminal care of adults is subcutaneous delivery [2] and this route is an attractive means of delivering the drug to children since it avoids intramuscular injections or the conventional continuous infusion, where access to, and the preservation of, small veins may be difficult [3]. Pharmacokinetic data for this means of delivering morphine has been obtained for adults [4] but not for children. In order to develop this type of protocol more fully, and assess the efficacy of the procedure it is necessary to obtain data on the concentrations of morphine and its metabolites in plasma following subcutaneous administration to children. The samples of blood that can be obtained from children during a pharmacokinetic study are necessarily small and limited by ethical constraints. Thus a sensitive and discriminating method was required in order to make multiple measurements of morphine and its metabolites in such small volumes of plasma.

Morphine is converted in the liver to its glucuronide metabolites and most of the morphine present in plasma, particularly after oral dosing, is in the form of its 3-glucuronide (M3G). The 6-glucuronide of morphine (M6G) is a potent analgesic [5, 6] and may also be present in plasma; at ca 10% of the concentration of M3G [5]. The amount of M3G in plasma following oral dosing is 10–50 times the amount of morphine, and thus M6G [6, 7] may be present in plasma in greater amounts than morphine.

A number of methods based on HPLC or GC–MS have been developed for the analysis of morphine [8–14]. Fewer methods have been developed for the analysis of the glucuronide metabolites of morphine, and the existing methods for the measurement of these compounds based on HPLC [7–11] are difficult to use and lack sensitivity; more sensitive methods have to be used for small volumes of samples. Recently, an elegant refinement of radioimmunoassay (RIA) technique has been described which was able to determine both morphine and M6G by using different antisera [15]. The method was validated using an established HPLC method. GC–MS methods cannot compete with RIA methods for speed but they are more specific than either HPLC or RIA methods.

---

* Author to whom correspondence should be addressed.

In this paper we describe a very sensitive and specific GC–MS method for measuring unconjugated morphine, codeine, normorphine and morphine as glucuronide(s) in small volumes of plasma from children.

Experimental

Chemicals

All solvents used were HPLC grade (Rathburn Chemicals, Peebleshire, UK). Chemicals and standards were obtained from the following sources: morphine sulphate pentahydrate, codeine free base, $[^2H_3]$ morphine, $[^2H_3]$ codeine, normorphine hydrochloride dihydrate, morphine 3-glucuronide, morphine 6-glucuronide dihydrate, glucuronidases from *Escherichia coli*, bovine liver, *Helix pomatia*, *Patella vulgata* and *Chlamys opercularis* (the Sigma Chemical Co., Dorset, UK); heptafluorobutyric anhydride (Aldrich Chemical Co., Dorset, UK).

Plasma samples

Morphine was infused subcutaneously at rates between 5 and 25 μg kg^{-1} h^{-1}. Samples of blood (1 ml) were collected at 4-h intervals from children receiving subcutaneous morphine infusion up to a total of 10 ml. The samples (up to a total of 1 ml kg^{-1} of body weight or 10 ml maximum regardless of body weight) were collected into a lithium heparin tube and then centrifuged, the plasma removed and the sample stored at $-20°C$ until analysis.

Treatment of samples

The volume of plasma obtained from 1 ml of blood was *ca* 0.5 ml. An aliquot of sample (300 μl) was withdrawn and to this were added 15 ng of $[^2H_3]$ morphine (15 μl of a 1 ng μl^{-1} solution in water) and 15 ng of $[^2H_3]$ codeine (15 μl of a 1 ng μl^{-1} solution in water).

(i) In order to determine unconjugated morphine in the spiked plasma sample two aliquots (each of 55 μl) were withdrawn and phosphate buffer (55 μl, 0.1 M, pH 6.8) was added to each, this was followed by addition of ammonia buffer (300 μl, 1 M, pH 9.5) and extraction with ethyl acetate (2 × 1 ml). The ethyl acetate was then removed under a stream of nitrogen and heptafluorobutyric anhydride (50 μl) was added to the residue. The solution was heated (15 min, 60°C), the reagent was then removed under a stream of nitrogen, the residue was dissolved in ethyl acetate (100 μl) and 4 μl were injected into the GC–MS.

(ii) In order to determine 3MG and 6MG the remaining plasma (220 μl) was mixed with phosphate buffer (220 μl, 0.1 M, pH 6.8) containing *E. coli* glucuronidase (2 mg ml^{-1}) and the mixture was then incubated at 42°C for 18 h. Two aliquots of 110-μl were withdrawn and treated as described in (i) starting from ". . . followed by addition of ammonia buffer . . .".

Calibration curve

The following solutions of standards were prepared

(a) $[^2H_3]$ morphine, $[^2H_3]$ codeine (each 1 ng μl^{-1}).

(b) Morphine, codeine and normorphine (0.05 ng μl^{-1}) + M3G and M6G (each 0.1 ng μl^{-1}).

(c) Morphine, codeine and normorphine (each 0.2 ng μl^{-1}) + M3G and M6G (each 0.4 ng μl^{-1}).

(d) Morphine, codeine and normorphine (each 0.8 ng μl^{-1}) + M3G and M6G (each 1.6 ng μl^{-1}).

(e) Morphine, codeine and normorphine (each 3.2 ng μl^{-1}).

Samples of plasma (300 μl) were spiked as follows;

(i) 15 μl of solution (a) + 15 μl of water;

(ii) 15 μl of solution (a) + 15 μl of solution (b);

(iii) 15 μl of solution (a) + 15 μl of solution (c);

(iv) 15 μl of solution (a) + 15 μl of solution (d);

(v) 15 μl of solution (a) + 15 μl of solution (e).

The spiked plasma samples (330 μl) were then treated as described under *Treatment of samples*.

Replicate precision

The following solutions of standards were prepared;

(a) $[^2H_3]$ morphine and $[^2H_3]$ codeine (each of 1 ng μl^{-1});

(b) Morphine, codeine and normorphine (each of 0.2 ng μl^{-1}) and M6G and M3G (each of 0.4 ng μl^{-1}).

A sample of blank plasma (1 ml) was spiked with 50 μl of solution (a) and 50 μl of solution (b) and mixed thoroughly.

(i) Five aliquots (each of 55 μl) were withdrawn and processed according to *Treatment of samples* (i).

(ii) The remaining plasma (0.825 ml) was mixed with phosphate buffer (0.825 ml, 0.1 M, pH 6.8) containing 2 mg ml^{-1} glucuronidase and the mixture was incubated at 42°C for 18 h. Five aliquots (each of 110 μl) were withdrawn and processed as previously aliquots described under *Treatment of samples.*

Instrumentation

A Hewlett–Packard 5998A GC–MS system was used. Analysis was carried out in the negative ion chemical ionization (NICI) mode. Methane was introduced to give a source pressure of *ca* 1 Torr. The GC was fitted with a Hewlett–Packard HP-1 column (12 m × 0.25 mm i.d. × 0.33 μm film), helium was used as a carrier gas with a head pressure of 5 p.s.i. The GC injector temperature was 250°C and the interface temperature was 280°C. The oven was programmed as follows: 100°C (1 min)/20°C min^{-1} to 250°C and then 2°C min^{-1} to 257°C. The mass spectrometer was tuned to the ions for the PFTBA calibrant at *m/z* 452, 595 and 633.

Results and Discussion

Figure 1 shows the mass spectrum of morphine di HFB derivative obtained under NICI conditions. The principal ions are the molecular ion at *m/z* 657, an ion at *m/z* 637 (resulting from loss of HF from the molecular ion), an ion at *m/z* 441 (due to a less straightforward fragmentation, probably involving addition of hydrogen followed by loss of HF and HFB) and a reagent specific ion (at *m/z* 197) which is the base peak. Selected ion monitoring was carried out for the ions at *m/z* 657 and *m/z* 637 in the analysis of morphine [^{2}H$_3$] morphine di HFB gave corresponding ions with the addition 3 a.m.u. HFB derivatives of normorphine and codeine also gave simple mass spectra under NICI conditions. Table 1 summarises the mass spectral and retention index data obtained for morphine and related compounds. Figure 2 shows an SIM trace for the HFB derivatives of a mixture of morphine, codeine and normorphine spiked at 0.38, 0.5 and 0.42 ng per 50 μl of plasma (the concentrations are expressed in terms of the free bases), respectively. The trace represents injection of *ca* 20 pg of each compound on column and these are compared with [^{2}H$_3$] morphine and [^{2}H$_3$] codeine spiked at 2.5 ng per 50 μl of plasma (*ca* 100 pg of each on column). The absolute limits of detection of the HFB derivatives of these compounds were below 1 pg.

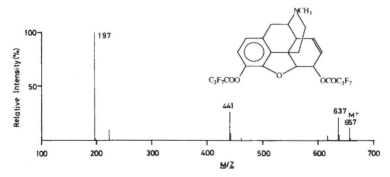

Figure 1
The mass spectrum of morphine diHFB derivative under NICI conditions.

Table 1
Mass spectral and chromatographic data

Compound	Base peak	M$^-$	Other major ions	*I* value
Morphine	197	657 (12.9)	637 (21.5), 441 (26.8)	2333
[^{2}H$_3$] morphine	214	660 (14.1)	640 (22.3), 444 (34.6)	2332
Codeine	475	475 (100)	213 (88.5)	2338
[^{2}H$_3$] codeine	478	478 (100)	213 (85.7)	2336
Normorphine	623	839 (7.8)	603 (34.7), 213 (56.8)	2404

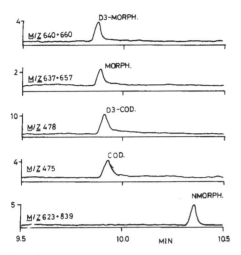

Figure 2
SIM trace showing the HFB derivatives of morphine, codeine and normorphine (0.2 ng per sample) in comparison with [^{2}H$_3$] morphine and codeine (2.5 ng per sample).

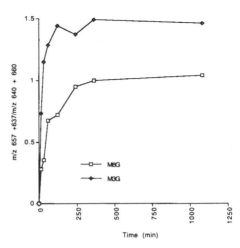

Figure 3
Release of morphine from M3G and M6G incubated with glucuronidase from *E. coli*.

Glucuronidases from *H. pomatia*, *P. vulgata*, *C. opercularis*, bovine liver and *E. coli* were tested for their ability to hydrolyse M3G and M6G and it was found that the *E. coli* glucuronidase was the most effective. The other enzymes gave <10% hydrolysis of the more readily hydrolysed M3G after 30 min. The *H. pomatia* enzyme has been used by a number of workers [16–18] and an early paper on its use [16] would seem to indicate that it only gives about 10% hydrolysis of M3G after 1 h whereas in our case the *E. coli* enzyme gave >80%. Acid hydrolysis has been commonly used to release morphine from its conjugates [14, 19], but here it was found that even mild acid hydrolysis led to extensive degradation. Typical curves for the hydrolysis of M3G and M6G by the *E. coli* glucuronidase are shown in Fig. 3. The hydrolysis of M3G was *ca* 70% complete in 30 min, whereas the hydrolysis of M6G was only *ca* 27% compete at this time. In principle, this provides a means of distinguishing between the two glucuronides but, in practice, the fact that M3G is 5–10 times more abundant that M6G in plasma [5] means that such a distinction is not possible within the limits of precision of the method.

The estimates for morphine as glucuronide are thus based on the curve constructed using morphine sulphate as a standard rather than curves constructed for the glucuronides. The

reason for this was that the commercial glucuronides were not pure as judged from the peak area for the morphine released after 18 h of hydrolysis compared to a calibration curve based on morphine sulphate, and the purities of M3G and M6G can be estimated as being *ca* 78 and 64%, respectively. It is not clear whether or not these standards have been fully authenticated and it is likely that they contain undefined amounts of absorbed water or exist in the form of more than one hydrate.

Calibration curves were constructed for morphine, codeine and normorphine by monitoring the selected ions for the compounds and deuterated internal standards given in Table 2. Normorphine was quantified against [^{2}H$_3$] morphine. The curves were constructed with respect to the compounds as their free bases and were linear over the following ranges: morphine 0.095–6.08 ng per 50 µl of plasma; codeine 0.125–8.0 ng per 50 µl of plasma; and normorphine 0.105–6.72 ng per 50 µl of plasma.

The precision and accuracy for the analysis of five samples of morphine (0.38 ng per 50 µl of plasma), codeine (0.5 ng per 50 µl of plasma) and normorphine (0.42 ng per 50 µl of plasma) was determined, and is shown in Table 3. The accuracy of the method was determined by comparing the amount of morphine, codeine or normorphine calculated from the

Table 2
Calibration curve details for morphine, codeine and normorphine

Compound	Ion ratio used to prepare curve	Equation of line	Corr. coeff.	Range ng per 50 μl
Morphine	$\dfrac{m/z\ 637\ +\ 657}{m/z\ 640\ +\ 660}$	$y = 1.2522x - 0.0143$	0.9998	0.095–6.08
Codeine	$\dfrac{m/z\ 475}{m/z\ 478}$	$y = 0.7044x - 0.0170$	0.9914	0.125–8.0
Normorphine	$\dfrac{m/z\ 839\ +\ 623}{m/z\ 640\ +\ 660}$	$y = 1.2536x - 0.2360$	0.9964	0.105–6.72

Table 3
Precision and accuracy of morphine, codeine and normofphine in subnanogram amounts

Compound	Amt spiked per 50 μl plasma	Accuracy $n = 5$	Precision $n = 5$
Morphine	0.38 ng	97.1%	±10.6%
M3G + M6G	0.8 ng each	—	±14.6%*
Codeine	0.5 ng	94.0%	±8.8%
Normorphine	0.42 ng	111.9%	±11.8%

* Determined after incubation for 18 h with glucuronidase.

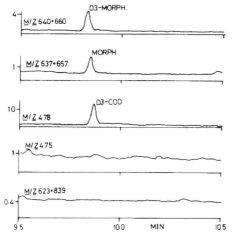

Figure 4
SIM trace showing morphine in a sample of plasma (50 μl) from a child receiving morphine via subcutaneous infusion for 24 h. Of [²H₃] morphine and codeine, 2.5 ng were added as internal standards.

The precision was quite good for determination of compounds at this level, the main source of imprecision was the difficulty of getting exactly reproducible integration with respect to the chromatographic baseline.

Figure 4 shows derivatized unconjugated morphine extracted from plasma (50 μl) following subcutaneous infusion of morphine for 24 h into a child comparison with standard derivatized [²H₃] morphine (2.5 ng per 50 μl). Figure 5 shows the same sample after treatment with glucuronidase for 18 h, indicating a large increase in the peak for morphine. After hydrolysis of the plasma samples with glucuronidase, it was possible to detect small amounts of normorphine. In some samples small amounts of codeine were detected at levels close to the limit of detection. Table 4 shows some preliminary results obtained after the analysis of plasma following the continuous

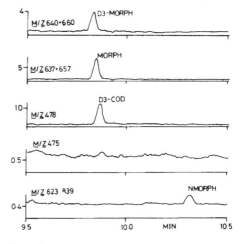

Figure 5
SIM trace showing morphine and normorphine in a sample of plasma (50 μl) from a child receiving morphine via subcutaneous infusion for 24 h. After hydrolysis with glucuronidase. Of [²H₃] morphine and codeine, 2.5 ng were added as internal standards.

analytical data using the calibration curve in comparison with the known amount of these compounds spiked into the sample. The precision of the analysis of M3G + M6G (0.8 ng per 50 μl of plasma) after incubation with glucuronidase for 18 h was determined, it was not possible to determine the accuracy in view of the doubts about the purity of the standards.

Table 4
The variation of the concentration of unconjugated and total morphine and total normorphine with time of subcutaneous infusion of morphine into children*

Time (h)	Patient 1			Patient 2†		
	Unconj. morphine (ng ml^{-1})	Total morphine (ng ml^{-1})	Total normorph. (ng ml^{-1})	Unconj. morphine (ng ml^{-1})	Total morphine (ng ml^{-1})	Total normorph. (ng ml^{-1})
0	4.72 ± 0.50	12.97 ± 0.47	ND‡	6.53	17.48	ND
4	4.48 ± 0.17	14.4 ± 0.76	ND	6.35	18.33	ND
8	—	—	—	3.82	13.77	ND
14	4.94 ± 0.21	39.78 ± 2.52	1.00 ± 0.50	—	—	—
18	6.73 ± 0.71	49.65 ± 0.72	0.89 ± 0.07	—	—	—
22	6.35 ± 0.10	58.1 ± 1.50	0.96 ± 0.12	5.74	41.18	1.37
24	5.24 ± 0.57	47.97 ± 0.88	0.96 ± 0.06	5.78 ± 0.24	47.18 ± 6.64	2.48 ± 0.72
26	5.44 ± 0.47	44.79 ± 2.89	0.88 ± 0.65	6.64	54.72	2.82
28	7.52 ± 0.32	58.54 ± 2.20	1.30 ± 0.23	5.62 ± 0.3	49.32 ± 6.48	2.67 ± 0.85

* Codeine was below the limit of detection (ca 0.25 ng ml^{-1}) in the 50-μl samples analysed.
† Some single measurements were made on samples from this patient.
‡ Not detected.

subcutaneous infusion of morphine (5–25 μg kg^{-1} h^{-1}) into children.

References

[1] S.E.F. Jones and M.A. Stokes, *Anaesthesia* **46**, 688–690 (1991).
[2] T.A. Goudie, M.W. Allan, M. Lonsdale, L.M. Burrow, W.A. Macrae and I.S. Grant, *Anaesthesia* **40**, 1086–1092 (1985).
[3] R. McNicol, *Br. J. Anaesth.* **71**, 752–756 (1993).
[4] C.S. Waldmann, J.R. Eason, E. Rambohul and G.C. Hanson, *Anaesthesia* **39**, 768–771 (1984).
[5] J. Sawe, J.O. Svensson and A. Rane, *Br. J. Clin. Pharmacol.* **16**, 85–93 (1983).
[6] R. Osbourne, S. Joel, D. Trew and M. Slevin, *Lancet* **I**, 828 (1988).
[7] R. Osbourne, P. Thompson, S. Joel, D. Trew, N. Patel and M. Slevin, *Br. J. Clin. Pharmacol.* **27**, 499–505 (1989).
[8] J.O. Svensson, A. Rane, J. Sawe and F. Sjoquist, *J. Chromatogr.* **230**, 427–432 (1982).

[9] J.O. Svensson, *J. Chromatogr.* **375** 174–178 (1986).
[10] P. Joel, R.J. Osborne and M. Slevin, *J. Chromatogr.* **430**, 394–399, (1988).
[11] R.F. Venn and A. Michalkiewicz, *J. Chromatogr.* **525**, 379–388 (1990).
[12] J.L. Mason, S.P. Ashmore and A.R. Aitkenhead, *J. Chromatogr.* **570**, 191–197 (1991).
[13] R.H. Drost, R.D. Van Ooijen, T. Ionescu and R.A.A. Maes, *J. Chromatogr.* **310**, 193–198 (1984).
[14] A.W. Jones, Y. Blom, U. Bondesson and E. Anggard, *J. Chromatogr.* **309**, 73–80 (1984).
[15] D.J. Chapman, S.P. Joel and G.W. Aherne, *J. Pharm. Biomed. Anal.* **12**, 353–360 (1994).
[16] D.B. Predmore, G.D. Christian and T.A. Loomis, *J. Forensic Sci.* **23**, 481–489 (1978).
[17] C. Lora-Tamayo, T. Tena and G. Tena, *J. Chromatogr.* **422**, 267–273 (1987).
[18] R. Wasels, F. Belleville, P. Paysant and P. Nabet, *J. Chromatogr.* **489**, 411–418 (1989).
[19] E.J. Cone, W.D. Darwin and W.F. Buchwald, *J. Chromatogr.* **275**, 307–318 (1983).

[Received for review 23 June 1994; revised manuscript received 15 August 1994]

JOURNAL OF
PHARMACEUTICAL
AND BIOMEDICAL
ANALYSIS

Journal of Pharmaceutical and Biomedical Analysis
29 (2002) 803–809

ELSEVIER

www.elsevier.com/locate/jpba

A simple microanalytical technique for the determination of paracetamol and its main metabolites in blood spots

E.J. Oliveira [a], D.G. Watson [a,*], N.S. Morton [b]

[a] *Department of Pharmaceutical Sciences, SIBS, University of Strathclyde, 27 Taylor Street, Glasgow G4 0NR, UK*
[b] *Department of Anaesthesiology, Royal Hospital for Sick Children, Yorkhill, Glasgow G3 8SJ, UK*

Received 27 December 2001; received in revised form 9 March 2002; accepted 30 March 2002

Abstract

The use of blood spot collection cards is a simple way to obtain specimens for analysis of drugs with a narrow therapeutic window. We describe the development and validation of a microanalytical technique for the determination of paracetamol and its glucuronide and sulphate metabolites from blood spots. The method is based on reversed phase high-performance liquid chromatography with ultraviolet detection. The limit of detection of the method is 600 pg on column for paracetamol. Intra- and inter-day precision of the determination of paracetamol was 7.1 and 3.2% respectively. The small volume of blood required (20 µl), combined with the simplicity of the analytical technique makes this a useful procedure for monitoring paracetamol concentrations. The method was applied to the analysis of blood spots taken from neonates being treated with paracetamol. © 2002 Elsevier Science B.V. All rights reserved.

Keywords: HPLC; Paracetamol; Paracetamol sulphate; Paracetamol glucuronide; Neonates

1. Introduction

Paracetamol (4-acetamidophenol) is the most used analgesic and antipyretic drug in children and neonates [1]. Despite its common use, pharmacokinetic data about paracetamol is scarce, especially in young infants and neonates. Due to differences in their metabolism, there is special interest in the levels of paracetamol in neonates, particularly after multiple dosing [2–4].

In neonates, the volume of blood taken is lim-

ited by ethical considerations and thus a method requiring only small volumes of blood is desirable. The use of a collection card similar to the Guthrie paper card used for the sampling of small volumes of blood allows more frequent sampling while still complying with ethical guidelines of a maximum 1 ml/kg body weight for blood sampling from neonates. This paper describes the development and validation of a microanalytical technique for the determination of paracetamol and its glucuronide and sulphate conjugates in blood spots. The technique is based on high-performance liquid chromatography (HPLC) with ultraviolet detection. Due to the general availability of liquid chromatographs coupled with the

* Corresponding author. Tel.: + 44-141-548-2651; fax: + 44-141-552-6443.
E-mail address: d.g.watson@strath.ac.uk (D.G. Watson).

0731-7085/02/$ - see front matter © 2002 Elsevier Science B.V. All rights reserved.
PII: S 0 7 3 1 - 7 0 8 5 (0 2) 0 0 1 7 4 - 7

simplicity of blood spot sampling the technique is well suited for the routine determination of blood levels of paracetamol and its main metabolites.

2. Materials and methods

2.1. Chemicals and reagents

Isolute ENV$^+$ solid phase extraction cartridges (3 ml, 500 mg) were purchased from IST (Mid Glamorgan, UK). Paracetamol and Hypersolv acetonitrile were obtained from BDH-Merck (Poole, Dorset, UK). Ammonium formate, 2-acetamidophenol and paracetamol glucuronide were purchased from Sigma-Aldrich (Poole, Dorset), and chlorosulfonic acid was purchased from Fluka (Poole, Dorset).

2.2. Paracetamol sulphate synthesis

Paracetamol sulphate was synthesised according to a published method [5]. The sulphate was purified by solid phase extraction using Isolute ENV$^+$ cartridges (3 ml, 500 mg). The cartridges were conditioned with 4 ml of methanol and 3 ml of water before loading the sample, which was dissolved in distilled water. The potassium chloride which was present in the paracetamol sulphate isolated from the reaction mixture was washed off with 3 ml of water and then the paracetamol sulphate was eluted with 6 ml (2 × 3 ml) of methanol. The procedure was repeated twice for the effluent collected during sample loading in order to recover any paracetamol sulphate which had not been retained during the first loading steps. Purity and identity of the paracetamol sulphate were confirmed by HPLC, electrospray mass spectrometry and ^{1}H and ^{13}C NMR data. NMR spectra were acquired on a Bruker AMX 400 MHz spectrometer using deuterated DMSO as the solvent and the positive ion electrospray mass spectrum on a Thermo-Finnigan Automass multi LC-GC/MS. High resolution fast atom bombardment mass spectrometry (FAB-MS) was carried out using a

JEOL 505HX instrument using the glycerol matrix as the calibrant.

^{1}H NMR (400 MHz, DMSO-d_6, δ from TMS): 1.99 (3H, s, COCH_3), 7.05 (2H, d, J = 8.76 Hz, H-3, H-5), 7.41 (2H, d, J = 8.84 Hz, H-2, H-6), 9.96 (1H, s, N–H). ^{13}C NMR (100 MHz, DMSO-d_6, δ from TMS): 168.80 (*C*OCH$_3$), 149.05 (C-4), 135.16 (C-1), 121.31 (C-2, C-6), 120.20 (C-3, C-5), 24.06 (COC*H*$_3$). Electrospray Mass Spectrometry: $m/z = 232$ [M + H]$^+$ base peak, m/z 151 [M-SO$_3$H]$^+$. FAB-MS gave the elemental composition of [M + H]$^+$ as: $C_8H_9NO_5S$ with an error of 2.4 ppm.

2.3. Sample collection preparation

Samples were taken from an indwelling arterial cannula placed for continuous blood pressure monitoring of neonates and infants in a paediatric intensive care unit. Single drops of blood were collected on Guthrie-type cards (Whatman, UK). For the purposes of calibration and development of the method drops of blood were taken from volunteers by finger-prick with a lancet. Paper discs (7 mm) were sampled from the blood spots with a hole puncher. The punched paper disks were transferred to 3.5 ml aluminium lined screw-capped vials and 200 µl of 20 mM ammonium formate buffer pH 3.5 was added. The samples were vortexed until blood was extracted from the paper (1–2 min). The internal standard (200 ng of 2-acetamidophenol) was added, and the samples were then mixed with 3 ml of acetonitrile. After brief vortexing to precipitate the proteins, samples were centrifuged (3500 × g for 5 min) and the supernatant transferred to another 3.5 ml vial. The solvent was evaporated to dryness under a stream of nitrogen and the residue was redissolved in 200 µl of 20 mM ammonium formate buffer pH 3.5. The sample was transferred to an autosampler vial fitted with a 200 µl glass insert and 20 µl was injected into the HPLC.

The volume of blood contained in the punched blood spot disks was determined by pipetting known volumes of blood (from 1 to 50 µl) onto the paper cards with an automatic pipette. The diameter of the blood spots were then measured and a calibration curve constructed. A power equation (see below) was fitted and the equation used to determine the volume of blood contained in the punched disks used for analysis, which had a fixed diameter of 7 mm. This procedure gave a figure of 15.84 μl of blood

Diameter of spot = 2.0624

$$\times \text{ volume of blood}^{0.4423}$$

$$(R^2 = 0.996).$$

The relationship between blood volume pipetted onto the cards and the diameter of the blood spot was linear from 10 to 50 μl. When a linear regression line was fitted between these points and the equation of the line used to calculate the volume of blood contained in 7 mm disks, the figure was 16.33 μl of blood. The volume of 16 μl of blood was thus used for calculating the paracetamol concentration in all the samples analysed.

2.4. Calibration solutions

Blood spots were collected from volunteers that were not receiving treatment with paracetamol. Punched paper disks were transferred to 3.5 ml aluminium lined screw-capped vials and solutions of standards (all prepared in acetonitrile) were spiked onto the paper discs. The solvent was evaporated to dryness under a stream of nitrogen and 200 μl of 20 mM ammonium formate buffer pH 3.5 was added. The samples were then extracted as described above for sample preparation.

2.5. HPLC analysis

HPLC was carried out using a Thermoseparations Spectra Series P4000 gradient pump coupled with a Spectra System UV 6000 LP photodiode array detector and a Thermoseparations AS1000 autosampler. The detector was set to scan from 200 to 500 nm and had a discrete channel set at 254 nm, which was the wavelength used for quantification. Separation was achieved using a Hypersil C18 column (75 × 4.6 mm, 3 μm). The mobile phase consisted of 20 mM ammonium formate buffer pH 3.5 (A) and methanol (B). The conditions of the gradient are specified in Table 1.

Precision of the method was estimated by analysing samples prepared by spiking blank blood spots with each analyte. The blood spots were extracted as described above for 'sample collection and preparation'. Intra-day precision was evaluated by analysing a series of samples prepared and analysed on the same day, while inter-day precision analyses were done with samples prepared and analysed on separate days (over a total period of 2 weeks). RSDs of less than 15% were considered satisfactory.

The limit of detection was based a peak height 3X the largest baseline fluctuation in mAu in a 1 min window around the elution time of the analyte in an analytical blank.

Recovery was calculated by comparing peak areas obtained for each analyte in samples prepared by spiking blank blood spots with peak areas obtained for samples of buffer spiked with

Table 1
Gradient conditions for HPLC analysis

Time (min)	20 mM ammonium formate pH 3.5 (%, v/v)	Methanol (%, v/v)	Flow (ml/min)
0.0	96.0	4.0	0.8
5.0	96.0	4.0	0.8
15.0	46.0	54.0	0.8
16.0	10.0	90.0	1.0
18.0	10.0	90.0	1.0
19.0	96.0	4.0	0.8
24.0	96.0	4.0	0.8

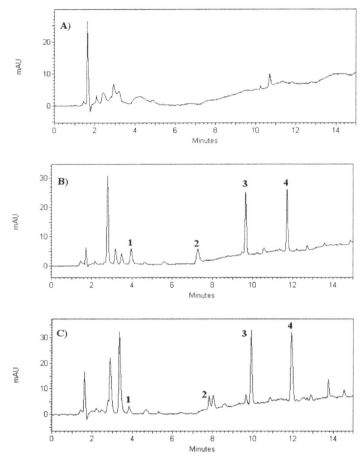

Fig. 1. HPLC chromatograms showing separation of the analytes. (A) Sample prepared from a blank bloodspot. (B) A calibration sample containing 600 ng/ml of paracetamol glucuronide (peak labelled 1), 600 ng/ml of paracetamol sulphate (peak labelled 2), and 300 ng/ml of paracetamol (peak labelled 3) extracted from a spiked blood spot. (C) A patient sample. The internal standard (2-acetamidophenol) is labelled as 4 in the chromatograms. Detection by UV at 254 nm. For HPLC gradient conditions see Table 1.

the same amount of the analytes. Paracetamol glucuronide and paracetamol sulphate were spiked at a concentration of 200 ng/ml, paracetamol was spiked at a concentration of 80 ng/ml, and 2-acetamidophenol at a concentration of 1 μg/ml. Recoveries above 80% were considered satisfactory.

3. Results

Fig. 1 shows chromatograms of a blank sample prepared from a blood spot (Fig. 1A), a calibration sample (Fig. 1B) prepared from a spiked blood spot and a sample from a patient (Fig. 1C). The chromatograms show that the analytes were well resolved from other endogenous components of plasma. The retention times were 3.88 ± 0.08 min for paracetamol glucuronide, 7.14 ± 0.18 min for paracetamol sulphate, 9.56 ± 0.05 min for paracetamol and 11.64 ± 0.05 min (mean $\pm$ S.D., $n = 5$) for 2-acetamidophenol (internal standard).

The response of the detector was linear for all the analytes (Table 2) over the concentration range used during analysis of samples. Since the detector response was lower for the metabolites of paracetamol compared to paracetamol itself, the limit of detection for paracetamol sulphate and paracetamol glucuronide (2 ng on column) was higher than that of paracetamol (600 pg on column).

The recovery of the analytes by the extraction procedure was estimated by comparing the peak area obtained for the analytes spiked in blank blood spot samples with the area of the analytes spiked in buffer (Table 3). The recovery was good and reproducible for paracetamol and the internal standard (2-acetamidophenol). The more variable recoveries obtained for the metabolites are possibly a consequence of their polar nature with correspondingly lower solubility in the extraction solvent. The recovery of paracetamol glucuronide was the most variable of all, which is a reflection of both its high polarity and its short retention time, which makes it more susceptible to interference from early eluting peaks.

The precision of the method (Table 4) was evaluated by analysing samples spiked with standards in concentrations close to the limit of detection. The samples were prepared and analysed on the same day (Intra-day precision), or prepared and analysed in different days (over a period of 2 weeks) for estimating inter-day precision. The precision was reasonable for a microanalytical method, and can possibly be im-

Table 2
Calibration curve parameters for paracetamol, paracetamol sulphate and paracetamol glucuronide

	Paracetamol glucuronide (mean, RSD, $n = 3$)	Paracetamol sulphate (mean, RSD, $n = 3$)	Paracetamol (mean, RSD, $n = 3$)
Slope	0.0005166, 10.7%	0.0007606, 3.1%	0.0028357, 7.3%
r^2	0.9978, 0.1%	0.9949, 0.6%	0.9973, 0.2%
Range (ng)	160–4000	160–4000	40–2000

Table 3
Recovery of the analytes by the extraction procedure

	Paracetamol glucuronide (%)	Paracetamol sulphate (%)	Paracetamol (%)	2-acetamidophenol (internal standard) (%)
Replicate 1	105.6	91.1	94.4	90.2
Replicate 2	90.9	76.0	93.9	86.9
Replicate 3	86.5	75.3	92.8	90.3
Replicate 4	106.4	88.4	96.5	90.6
Replicate 5	96.08	100.3	92.6	99.2
Replicate 6	66.13	73.6	93.1	91.3
Average	91.9	84.1	93.9	91.5
RSD%	16.2	12.8	1.5	4.5

Values are percentage of recovery when compared with the average peak area of the analytes spiked in buffer. Paracetamol glucuronide and paracetamol sulphate were spiked at a concentration of 200 ng/ml, paracetamol was spiked at a concentration of 80 ng/ml, and 2-acetamidophenol at a concentration of 1 μg/ml.

Table 4
Intra- and inter-day precision of the method

	Paracetamol glucuronide (ng/ml)	Paracetamol sulphate (ng/ml)	Paracetamol (ng/ml)
Intra-day precision			
Replicate 1	145.3	160.5	39.9
Replicate 2	151.2	134.8	46.4
Replicate 3	150.7	142.1	41.6
Replicate 4	165.0	139.8	46.8
Replicate 5	155.2	190.1	42.2
Average	153.5	153.5	43.4
RSD%	4.8	14.8	7.1
Inter-day precision			
Replicate 1	162.9	126.4	42.1
Replicate 2	182.9	139.8	43.6
Replicate 3	209.9	132.2	41.2
Replicate 4	174.1	169.2	40.4
Average	182.4	141.9	41.8
RSD%	11.0	13.4	3.2

The samples were spiked with a nominal concentration of 160 ng/ml for paracetamol glucuronide, 160 ng/ml of paracetamol sulphate, and 40 ng/ml of paracetamol.

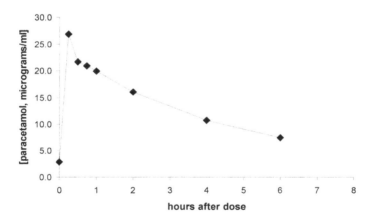

Fig. 2. Time profile of paracetamol concentration in blood spots taken from a neonate after a rectal dose of 20 mg/kg.

proved if a larger volume of sample were injected or if the sample was prepared in more concentrated form (for example by diluting it to a final volume of 100 µl, instead of 200 µl).

An example of the application of this method to the determination of paracetamol concentrations in blood spots from neonates is shown in Fig. 2.

4. Discussion

Although widely used as an analgesic and antipyretic, the pharmacokinetics of paracetamol in young infants and neonates is not fully understood. There are reports that paracetamol administered rectally in neonates at a dose of 20 mg/kg body weight results in subtherapeutic concentrations [2,3]. Neonates are known to have a different metabolic profile, and in the case of paracetamol, sulphation is known to be the major route for metabolism [4]. A better understanding of the pharmacokinetics of paracetamol in neonates is necessary to ensure that paracetamol plasma concentrations do not reach toxic or fall to subtherapeutic levels, especially when multiple dosing is being used. The development of sensitive and selective methods for measuring paracetamol concentrations in biological fluids is an important prerequisite of this endeavour.

Most methods for determining paracetamol in biological samples use HPLC [6–8] or gas-chromatography [9–11]. Other methods include enzymatic and colorimetric techniques. Methods that use a small volume of blood are desirable in situations where the collection of larger volumes are not feasible, such as in the case of neonates, for which the volume of blood sampled is limited by ethical guidelines. Also, other features which are desirable are simplicity of sample preparation and general availability of the analytical instrument required for analysis. A recent method [12] makes use of only 10 µl of blood or plasma and relies on HPLC with electrochemical detection for quantification of paracetamol. The method described here makes use of HPLC with ultraviolet detection, which is widely available in biochemical laboratories. It has the advantage of requiring only a small sample volume (20 µl) combined with simple sample preparation and analysis. The analytes are well resolved from endogenous components from the blood (Fig. 1) and the method can be applied to detection of paracetamol and its metabolites. The short retention time of paracetamol glucuronide means that it is the analyte most prone to suffer interference from polar components eluting early in the run. However, in most cases resolution from interfering peaks was achieved. The use of new reversed phase columns that can run 100% aqueous mobile phases (through the use of stationary phases with polar end-capping functionalities) might improve retention of the glucuronide and improve precision of the method for this analyte.

Acknowledgements

This work was supported by a British Journal of Anaesthesia/Royal College of Anaesthetists grant, we also thank the Wellcome Trust for Support and Dr Sandy Gray (Strathclyde University) for the acquisition of NMR data.

References

[1] A. Arana, N.S. Morton, T.G. Hansen, Acta Anaesthesiologica Scandinavica 45 (2001) 20–29.
[2] T.G. Hansen, K. O'Brien, N.S. Morton, S.N. Rasmussen, Acta Anaesthesiologica Scandinavica 43 (1999) 855–859.
[3] Y.C. Lin, H. Sussman, W. Benitz, Paediatric Anaesthesia 7 (1997) 457–459.
[4] R.A. Van Lingen, J.T. Deinum, J.M.E. Quak, A.J. Kuizenga, J.G. Van Dam, K.J.S. Anand, D. Tibboel, A. Okken, Archives of Disease in Childhood: Fetal and Neonatal Edition 80 (1999) F59–F63.
[5] J. Feigenbaum, C.A. Neuberg, Journal of the American Chemical Society 63 (1941) 3529–3530.
[6] V. Bari, U.J. Dhorda, M. Sundaresan, Indian Drugs 35 (1998) 222–225.
[7] A.G. Goicoechea, M.J. Lopez De Alda, J.L. Vila-Jato, Journal of Liquid Chromatography 18 (1995) 3257–3268.
[8] E. Pufal, M. Sykutera, G. Rochholz, H.W. Schutz, K. Sliwka, H.J. Kaatsch, Fresenius Journal of Analytical Chemistry 367 (2000) 596–599.
[9] K. Chan, J.F. McCann, Journal of Chromatography 164 (1979) 394–398.
[10] E. Kaa, Journal of Chromatography 221 (1980) 414–418.
[11] D.J. Speed, S.J. Dickson, E.R. Cairns, N.D. Kim, Journal of Analytical Toxicology 25 (2001) 198–202.
[12] R. Whelpton, K. Fernandes, K.A. Wilkinson, D.R. Goldhill, Biomedical Chromatography 7 (1993) 90–93.

ELSEVIER

Journal of Pharmaceutical and Biomedical Analysis
29 (2002) 803–809

JOURNAL OF
PHARMACEUTICAL
AND BIOMEDICAL
ANALYSIS

www.elsevier.com/locate/jpba

A simple microanalytical technique for the determination of paracetamol and its main metabolites in blood spots

E.J. Oliveira [a], D.G. Watson [a,*], N.S. Morton [b]

[a] *Department of Pharmaceutical Sciences, SIBS, University of Strathclyde, 27 Taylor Street, Glasgow G4 0NR, UK*
[b] *Department of Anaesthesiology, Royal Hospital for Sick Children, Yorkhill, Glasgow G3 8SJ, UK*

Received 27 December 2001; received in revised form 9 March 2002; accepted 30 March 2002

Abstract

The use of blood spot collection cards is a simple way to obtain specimens for analysis of drugs with a narrow therapeutic window. We describe the development and validation of a microanalytical technique for the determination of paracetamol and its glucuronide and sulphate metabolites from blood spots. The method is based on reversed phase high-performance liquid chromatography with ultraviolet detection. The limit of detection of the method is 600 pg on column for paracetamol. Intra- and inter-day precision of the determination of paracetamol was 7.1 and 3.2% respectively. The small volume of blood required (20 μl), combined with the simplicity of the analytical technique makes this a useful procedure for monitoring paracetamol concentrations. The method was applied to the analysis of blood spots taken from neonates being treated with paracetamol. © 2002 Elsevier Science B.V. All rights reserved.

Keywords: HPLC; Paracetamol; Paracetamol sulphate; Paracetamol glucuronide; Neonates

1. Introduction

Paracetamol (4-acetamidophenol) is the most used analgesic and antipyretic drug in children and neonates [1]. Despite its common use, pharmacokinetic data about paracetamol is scarce, especially in young infants and neonates. Due to differences in their metabolism, there is special interest in the levels of paracetamol in neonates, particularly after multiple dosing [2–4].

In neonates, the volume of blood taken is lim-

ited by ethical considerations and thus a method requiring only small volumes of blood is desirable. The use of a collection card similar to the Guthrie paper card used for the sampling of small volumes of blood allows more frequent sampling while still complying with ethical guidelines of a maximum 1 ml/kg body weight for blood sampling from neonates. This paper describes the development and validation of a microanalytical technique for the determination of paracetamol and its glucuronide and sulphate conjugates in blood spots. The technique is based on high-performance liquid chromatography (HPLC) with ultraviolet detection. Due to the general availability of liquid chromatographs coupled with the

---

* Corresponding author. Tel.: + 44-141-548-2651; fax: + 44-141-552-6443.
E-mail address: d.g.watson@strath.ac.uk (D.G. Watson).

0731-7085/02/$ - see front matter © 2002 Elsevier Science B.V. All rights reserved.
PII: S 0 7 3 1 - 7 0 8 5 (0 2) 0 0 1 7 4 - 7

simplicity of blood spot sampling the technique is well suited for the routine determination of blood levels of paracetamol and its main metabolites.

2. Materials and methods

2.1. Chemicals and reagents

Isolute ENV$^+$ solid phase extraction cartridges (3 ml, 500 mg) were purchased from IST (Mid Glamorgan, UK). Paracetamol and Hypersolv acetonitrile were obtained from BDH-Merck (Poole, Dorset, UK). Ammonium formate, 2-acetamidophenol and paracetamol glucuronide were purchased from Sigma-Aldrich (Poole, Dorset), and chlorosulfonic acid was purchased from Fluka (Poole, Dorset).

2.2. Paracetamol sulphate synthesis

Paracetamol sulphate was synthesised according to a published method [5]. The sulphate was purified by solid phase extraction using Isolute ENV$^+$ cartridges (3 ml, 500 mg). The cartridges were conditioned with 4 ml of methanol and 3 ml of water before loading the sample, which was dissolved in distilled water. The potassium chloride which was present in the paracetamol sulphate isolated from the reaction mixture was washed off with 3 ml of water and then the paracetamol sulphate was eluted with 6 ml (2 × 3 ml) of methanol. The procedure was repeated twice for the effluent collected during sample loading in order to recover any paracetamol sulphate which had not been retained during the first loading steps. Purity and identity of the paracetamol sulphate were confirmed by HPLC, electrospray mass spectrometry and ^{1}H and ^{13}C NMR data. NMR spectra were acquired on a Bruker AMX 400 MHz spectrometer using deuterated DMSO as the solvent and the positive ion electrospray mass spectrum on a Thermo-Finnigan Automass multi LC-GC/MS. High resolution fast atom bombardment mass spectrometry (FAB-MS) was carried out using a

JEOL 505HX instrument using the glycerol matrix as the calibrant.

^{1}H NMR (400 MHz, DMSO-d_6, δ from TMS): 1.99 (3H, s, COCH_3), 7.05 (2H, d, J = 8.76 Hz, H-3, H-5), 7.41 (2H, d, J = 8.84 Hz, H-2, H-6), 9.96 (1H, s, N–H). ^{13}C NMR (100 MHz, DMSO-d_6, δ from TMS): 168.80 (COCH$_3$), 149.05 (C-4), 135.16 (C-1), 121.31 (C-2, C-6), 120.20 (C-3, C-5), 24.06 (COCH$_3$). Electrospray Mass Spectrometry: m/z = 232 [M + H]$^+$ base peak, m/z 151 [M-SO$_3$H]$^+$. FAB-MS gave the elemental composition of [M + H]$^+$ as: $C_8H_9NO_5S$ with an error of 2.4 ppm.

2.3. Sample collection preparation

Samples were taken from an indwelling arterial cannula placed for continuous blood pressure monitoring of neonates and infants in a paediatric intensive care unit. Single drops of blood were collected on Guthrie-type cards (Whatman, UK). For the purposes of calibration and development of the method drops of blood were taken from volunteers by finger-prick with a lancet. Paper discs (7 mm) were sampled from the blood spots with a hole puncher. The punched paper disks were transferred to 3.5 ml aluminium lined screw-capped vials and 200 μl of 20 mM ammonium formate buffer pH 3.5 was added. The samples were vortexed until blood was extracted from the paper (1–2 min). The internal standard (200 ng of 2-acetamidophenol) was added, and the samples were then mixed with 3 ml of acetonitrile. After brief vortexing to precipitate the proteins, samples were centrifuged (3500 × g for 5 min) and the supernatant transferred to another 3.5 ml vial. The solvent was evaporated to dryness under a stream of nitrogen and the residue was redissolved in 200 μl of 20 mM ammonium formate buffer pH 3.5. The sample was transferred to an autosampler vial fitted with a 200 μl glass insert and 20 μl was injected into the HPLC.

The volume of blood contained in the punched blood spot disks was determined by pipetting known volumes of blood (from 1 to 50 μl) onto the paper cards with an automatic pipette. The diameter of the blood spots were then measured and a calibration curve constructed. A power equation (see below) was fitted and the equation used to determine the volume of blood contained in the punched disks used for analysis, which had a fixed diameter of 7 mm. This procedure gave a figure of 15.84 µl of blood

Diameter of spot = 2.0624

$$\times \text{ volume of blood}^{0.4423}$$

$$(R^2 = 0.996).$$

The relationship between blood volume pipetted onto the cards and the diameter of the blood spot was linear from 10 to 50 µl. When a linear regression line was fitted between these points and the equation of the line used to calculate the volume of blood contained in 7 mm disks, the figure was 16.33 µl of blood. The volume of 16 µl of blood was thus used for calculating the paracetamol concentration in all the samples analysed.

2.4. Calibration solutions

Blood spots were collected from volunteers that were not receiving treatment with paracetamol. Punched paper disks were transferred to 3.5 ml aluminium lined screw-capped vials and solutions of standards (all prepared in acetonitrile) were spiked onto the paper discs. The solvent was evaporated to dryness under a stream of nitrogen and 200 µl of 20 mM ammonium formate buffer pH 3.5 was added. The samples were then extracted as described above for sample preparation.

2.5. HPLC analysis

HPLC was carried out using a Thermoseparations Spectra Series P4000 gradient pump coupled with a Spectra System UV 6000 LP photodiode array detector and a Thermoseparations AS1000 autosampler. The detector was set to scan from 200 to 500 nm and had a discrete channel set at 254 nm, which was the wavelength used for quantification. Separation was achieved using a Hypersil C18 column (75 × 4.6 mm, 3 µm). The mobile phase consisted of 20 mM ammonium formate buffer pH 3.5 (A) and methanol (B). The conditions of the gradient are specified in Table 1.

Precision of the method was estimated by analysing samples prepared by spiking blank blood spots with each analyte. The blood spots were extracted as described above for 'sample collection and preparation'. Intra-day precision was evaluated by analysing a series of samples prepared and analysed on the same day, while inter-day precision analyses were done with samples prepared and analysed on separate days (over a total period of 2 weeks). RSDs of less than 15% were considered satisfactory.

The limit of detection was based a peak height 3X the largest baseline fluctuation in mAu in a 1 min window around the elution time of the analyte in an analytical blank.

Recovery was calculated by comparing peak areas obtained for each analyte in samples prepared by spiking blank blood spots with peak areas obtained for samples of buffer spiked with

Table 1
Gradient conditions for HPLC analysis

Time (min)	20 mM ammonium formate pH 3.5 (%, v/v)	Methanol (%, v/v)	Flow (ml/min)
0.0	96.0	4.0	0.8
5.0	96.0	4.0	0.8
15.0	46.0	54.0	0.8
16.0	10.0	90.0	1.0
18.0	10.0	90.0	1.0
19.0	96.0	4.0	0.8
24.0	96.0	4.0	0.8

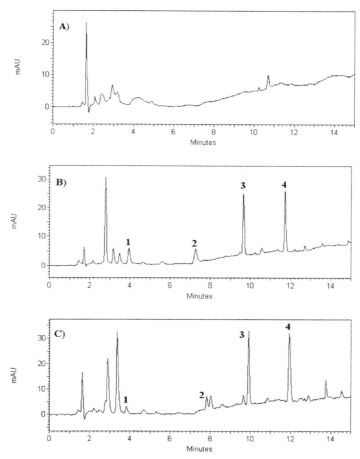

Fig. 1. HPLC chromatograms showing separation of the analytes. (A) Sample prepared from a blank bloodspot. (B) A calibration sample containing 600 ng/ml of paracetamol glucuronide (peak labelled 1), 600 ng/ml of paracetamol sulphate (peak labelled 2), and 300 ng/ml of paracetamol (peak labelled 3) extracted from a spiked blood spot. (C) A patient sample. The internal standard (2-acetamidophenol) is labelled as 4 in the chromatograms. Detection by UV at 254 nm. For HPLC gradient conditions see Table 1.

the same amount of the analytes. Paracetamol glucuronide and paracetamol sulphate were spiked at a concentration of 200 ng/ml, paracetamol was spiked at a concentration of 80 ng/ml, and 2-acetamidophenol at a concentration of 1 µg/ml. Recoveries above 80% were considered satisfactory.

3. Results

Fig. 1 shows chromatograms of a blank sample prepared from a blood spot (Fig. 1A), a calibration sample (Fig. 1B) prepared from a spiked blood spot and a sample from a patient (Fig. 1C). The chromatograms show that the analytes were well resolved from other endogenous components of plasma. The retention times were 3.88 ± 0.08 min for paracetamol glucuronide, 7.14 ± 0.18 min for paracetamol sulphate, 9.56 ± 0.05 min for paracetamol and 11.64 ± 0.05 min (mean $\pm$ S.D., $n = 5$) for 2-acetamidophenol (internal standard).

The response of the detector was linear for all the analytes (Table 2) over the concentration range used during analysis of samples. Since the detector response was lower for the metabolites of paracetamol compared to paracetamol itself, the limit of detection for paracetamol sulphate and paracetamol glucuronide (2 ng on column) was higher than that of paracetamol (600 pg on column).

The recovery of the analytes by the extraction procedure was estimated by comparing the peak area obtained for the analytes spiked in blank blood spot samples with the area of the analytes spiked in buffer (Table 3). The recovery was good and reproducible for paracetamol and the internal standard (2-acetamidophenol). The more variable recoveries obtained for the metabolites are possibly a consequence of their polar nature with correspondingly lower solubility in the extraction solvent. The recovery of paracetamol glucuronide was the most variable of all, which is a reflection of both its high polarity and its short retention time, which makes it more susceptible to interference from early eluting peaks.

The precision of the method (Table 4) was evaluated by analysing samples spiked with standards in concentrations close to the limit of detection. The samples were prepared and analysed on the same day (Intra-day precision), or prepared and analysed in different days (over a period of 2 weeks) for estimating inter-day precision. The precision was reasonable for a microanalytical method, and can possibly be im-

Table 2
Calibration curve parameters for paracetamol, paracetamol sulphate and paracetamol glucuronide

	Paracetamol glucuronide (mean, RSD, $n = 3$)	Paracetamol sulphate (mean, RSD, $n = 3$)	Paracetamol (mean, RSD, $n = 3$)
Slope	0.0005166, 10.7%	0.0007606, 3.1%	0.0028357, 7.3%
r^2	0.9978, 0.1%	0.9949, 0.6%	0.9973, 0.2%
Range (ng)	160–4000	160–4000	40–2000

Table 3
Recovery of the analytes by the extraction procedure

	Paracetamol glucuronide (%)	Paracetamol sulphate (%)	Paracetamol (%)	2-acetamidophenol (internal standard) (%)
Replicate 1	105.6	91.1	94.4	90.2
Replicate 2	90.9	76.0	93.9	86.9
Replicate 3	86.5	75.3	92.8	90.3
Replicate 4	106.4	88.4	96.5	90.6
Replicate 5	96.08	100.3	92.6	99.2
Replicate 6	66.13	73.6	93.1	91.3
Average	91.9	84.1	93.9	91.5
RSD%	16.2	12.8	1.5	4.5

Values are percentage of recovery when compared with the average peak area of the analytes spiked in buffer. Paracetamol glucuronide and paracetamol sulphate were spiked at a concentration of 200 ng/ml, paracetamol was spiked at a concentration of 80 ng/ml, and 2-acetamidophenol at a concentration of 1 μg/ml.

Table 4
Intra- and inter-day precision of the method

	Paracetamol glucuronide (ng/ml)	Paracetamol sulphate (ng/ml)	Paracetamol (ng/ml)
Intra-day precision			
Replicate 1	145.3	160.5	39.9
Replicate 2	151.2	134.8	46.4
Replicate 3	150.7	142.1	41.6
Replicate 4	165.0	139.8	46.8
Replicate 5	155.2	190.1	42.2
Average	153.5	153.5	43.4
RSD%	4.8	14.8	7.1
Inter-day precision			
Replicate 1	162.9	126.4	42.1
Replicate 2	182.9	139.8	43.6
Replicate 3	209.9	132.2	41.2
Replicate 4	174.1	169.2	40.4
Average	182.4	141.9	41.8
RSD%	11.0	13.4	3.2

The samples were spiked with a nominal concentration of 160 ng/ml for paracetamol glucuronide, 160 ng/ml of paracetamol sulphate, and 40 ng/ml of paracetamol.

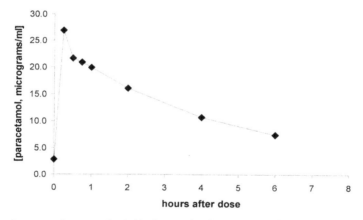

Fig. 2. Time profile of paracetamol concentration in blood spots taken from a neonate after a rectal dose of 20 mg/kg.

proved if a larger volume of sample were injected or if the sample was prepared in more concentrated form (for example by diluting it to a final volume of 100 μl, instead of 200 μl).

An example of the application of this method to the determination of paracetamol concentrations in blood spots from neonates is shown in Fig. 2.

4. Discussion

Although widely used as an analgesic and antipyretic, the pharmacokinetics of paracetamol in young infants and neonates is not fully understood. There are reports that paracetamol administered rectally in neonates at a dose of 20 mg/kg body weight results in subtherapeutic concentrations [2,3]. Neonates are known to have a different metabolic profile, and in the case of paracetamol, sulphation is known to be the major route for metabolism [4]. A better understanding of the pharmacokinetics of paracetamol in neonates is necessary to ensure that paracetamol plasma concentrations do not reach toxic or fall to subtherapeutic levels, especially when multiple dosing is being used. The development of sensitive and selective methods for measuring paracetamol concentrations in biological fluids is an important prerequisite of this endeavour.

Most methods for determining paracetamol in biological samples use HPLC [6–8] or gas-chromatography [9–11]. Other methods include enzymatic and colorimetric techniques. Methods that use a small volume of blood are desirable in situations where the collection of larger volumes are not feasible, such as in the case of neonates, for which the volume of blood sampled is limited by ethical guidelines. Also, other features which are desirable are simplicity of sample preparation and general availability of the analytical instrument required for analysis. A recent method [12] makes use of only 10 μl of blood or plasma and relies on HPLC with electrochemical detection for quantification of paracetamol. The method described here makes use of HPLC with ultraviolet detection, which is widely available in biochemical laboratories. It has the advantage of requiring only a small sample volume (20 μl) combined with simple sample preparation and analysis. The analytes are well resolved from endogenous components from the blood (Fig. 1) and the method can be applied to detection of paracetamol and its metabolites. The short retention time of paracetamol glucuronide means that it is the analyte most prone to suffer interference from polar components eluting early in the run. However, in most cases resolution from interfering peaks was

achieved. The use of new reversed phase columns that can run 100% aqueous mobile phases (through the use of stationary phases with polar end-capping functionalities) might improve retention of the glucuronide and improve precision of the method for this analyte.

Acknowledgements

This work was supported by a British Journal of Anaesthesia/Royal College of Anaesthetists grant, we also thank the Wellcome Trust for Support and Dr Sandy Gray (Strathclyde University) for the acquisition of NMR data.

References

[1] A. Arana, N.S. Morton, T.G. Hansen, Acta Anaesthesiologica Scandinavica 45 (2001) 20–29.
[2] T.G. Hansen, K. O'Brien, N.S. Morton, S.N. Rasmussen, Acta Anaesthesiologica Scandinavica 43 (1999) 855–859.
[3] Y.C. Lin, H. Sussman, W. Benitz, Paediatric Anaesthesia 7 (1997) 457–459.
[4] R.A. Van Lingen, J.T. Deinum, J.M.E. Quak, A.J. Kuizenga, J.G. Van Dam, K.J.S. Anand, D. Tibboel, A. Okken, Archives of Disease in Childhood: Fetal and Neonatal Edition 80 (1999) F59–F63.
[5] J. Feigenbaum, C.A. Neuberg, Journal of the American Chemical Society 63 (1941) 3529–3530.
[6] V. Bari, U.J. Dhorda, M. Sundaresan, Indian Drugs 35 (1998) 222–225.
[7] A.G. Goicoechea, M.J. Lopez De Alda, J.L. Vila-Jato, Journal of Liquid Chromatography 18 (1995) 3257–3268.
[8] E. Pufal, M. Sykutera, G. Rochholz, H.W. Schutz, K. Sliwka, H.J. Kaatsch, Fresenius Journal of Analytical Chemistry 367 (2000) 596–599.
[9] K. Chan, J.F. McCann, Journal of Chromatography 164 (1979) 394–398.
[10] E. Kaa, Journal of Chromatography 221 (1980) 414–418.
[11] D.J. Speed, S.J. Dickson, E.R. Cairns, N.D. Kim, Journal of Analytical Toxicology 25 (2001) 198–202.
[12] R. Whelpton, K. Fernandes, K.A. Wilkinson, D.R. Goldhill, Biomedical Chromatography 7 (1993) 90–93.

Full Text

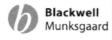 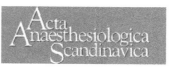

Plasma concentrations and pharmacokinetics of bupivacaine with and without adrenaline following caudal anaesthesia in infants

Author(s):	Hansen, T. G[1]; Morton, N. S[1]; Cullen, P. M[1]; Watson, D. G[2]
Issue:	Volume 45(1), January 2001, pp 42-47
Publication Type:	[Regional Anaesthesia & Pain Therapy]
Publisher:	© 2001 The Acta Anaesthesiologica Foundation.
Institution(s):	[1]Directorate of Anaesthesia, The Royal Hospital for Sick Children, Yorkhill, Glasgow, and [2]Department of Pharmaceutical Sciences, University of Strathclyde, Glasgow, Scotland, United Kingdom
	Received 31 January, accepted for publication 29 June 2000
	Address: Dr. Tom G. Hansen; Department of Anaesthesia & Intensive Care; Odense University Hospital; DK-5000 Odense; Denmark; e-mail: tomghansen@dadlnet.dk

ISSN: 0001-5172
Accession: 11152032

Keywords: Algorithms, Anesthesia, Epidural, Anesthetics, Local, Anesthetics, Local, Bupivacaine, Bupivacaine, Epidural Space, Epinephrine, Half-Life, Humans, Infant, Vasoconstrictor Agents

Abstract

Background: The aim of this study was to determine whether the use of adrenaline 1/400 000 added to 0.25% bupivacaine significantly delays the systemic absorption of the drug from the caudal epidural space in young infants.

Methods: Fifteen infants less than 5 months of age undergoing minor lower abdominal procedures under a standardised general anaesthetic were randomised to receive a caudal block with either 0.25% plain bupivacaine 2.5 mg/kg (n=7) or bupivacaine 0.25% with 1/400 000 adrenaline (n=8). Blood samples were drawn at 30, 60, 90, 180, 240 and 360 min according to the infant's weight and analysed for total and free bupivacaine concentrations using a gas chromatography-mass spectrometry (GC-MS) technique.

Results: The total C_{MAX} and T_{MAX} were comparable in both groups. The total bupivacaine concentration at t=360 min was significantly higher in the "adrenaline" group compared to the "plain" group, i.e. a median (range) 742 ng/ml (372-1423 ng/ml) vs. 400.5 ng/ml (114-446 ng/ml), P=0.0080. The median "apparent" terminal half-life (t1/2) was significantly longer in the "adrenaline" group (363 min; range 238-537 min) compared to the "plain" group (n=6) (165 min; range 104-264 min), P=0.0087. The free bupivacaine concentrations (n=3 in both groups) ranged between 13 ng/ml and 52 ng/ml, corresponding to a percentage of free bupivacaine between 1.3% and 6.7%.

Conclusion: The addition of 1/400.000 adrenaline prolongs the systemic absorption of caudally administered bupivacaine in infants less than 5 months of age.

Caudal epidural block with bupivacaine is by far the commonest regional anaesthetic technique used in small children (1-3). It combines the advantages of a fairly simple technique with a high success rate. The pharmacokinetics of caudally administered bupivacaine in young children, however, is still relatively little known (4-8).

The plasma protein binding capacity in infants is decreased (5, 9). This is an important issue when using highly plasma protein bound drugs such as bupivacaine. This reduction in binding capacity for bupivacaine will increase the free unbound fraction in infants, and thus increase the possibilities of toxic effects.

The "toxic" free plasma bupivacaine concentration following a single caudal bupivacaine dose is currently not known, but central nervous system toxicity in both adults and children has been described at total plasma bupivacaine concentrations in excess of 2 µg/ml (10).

By adding adrenaline to the bupivacaine solution it has been claimed that the systemic absorption of caudally (epidural) administered bupivacaine can be lowered considerably. Clinically, however, the addition of 1/200 000 adrenaline to 0.25% bupivacaine has been found both to prolong the duration of the block (11) and to have no effects at all (12).

The aim of this study was to determine whether the use of adrenaline 1/400 000 added to 0.25% bupivacaine significantly delays the systemic absorption of the drug from the caudal epidural space in young infants.

Methods

Following ethical approval and written informed parental consent, 15 infants less than 5 months of age scheduled for minor lower abdominal surgery were enrolled in this study. Infants with any known renal or hepatic impairments were excluded as were infants suffering from contraindications to caudal anaesthesia. Preoperatively, the infants were randomised to receive a caudal block with either plain 0.25% bupivacaine (n=7) or 0.25% bupivacaine with adrenaline (1/400 000) (n=8). Sequential numbered opaque and sealed envelopes carried out randomisation. The total volume of 0.25% bupivacaine (with or without adrenaline) in each group was 1 ml/kg (=2.5 mg/kg).

Anaesthetic technique

Apart from the topical application of EMLA cream, no premedication was given. All infants received a standardised non-opioid-based general anaesthetic technique comprising induction with thiopenthone (3-5 mg/kg) and atracurium (0.5 mg/kg). Following endotracheal intubation, the infants were ventilated to normocapnia with 40% O_2 in N_2O and desflurane (6-10%).

Subsequently, the infants were placed in the left lateral position and the caudal block performed using an aseptic technique and a 23 G needle. When negative aspiration of blood or cerebrospinal fluid had been confirmed, the calculated dose of bupivacaine (± adrenaline) was injected slowly and in increments into the caudal space while watching vital signs and the electrocardiographic (ECG) monitor.

After surgery, residual neuromuscular blockade was reversed with glycopyrrolate (10 µg/kg) and neostigmine (50 µg/kg) and all children were extubated.

Blood sampling

Following the anaesthetic induction, a dedicated peripheral intravenous cannula (Venflon 22 G, Ohmeda, Sweden) was inserted in a saphenous vein for blood sampling. Patency of this cannula was maintained by an infusion of 5% glucose with 0.225% saline 3-5 ml/h.

Blood samples (0.7-1.0 ml/sample) were collected from the cannula at 30, 60, 90, 180, 240 and 360 min after the caudal block. After each blood sample the i.v. catheter was flushed with heparinised saline. The total number of blood samples from each individual was restricted by the Ethics Committee's limit of 1 ml/kg, but it was possible to sample from all but one infant at 30, 60 and 360 min. Older infants had additional samples drawn at intermediate time points according to weight.

The blood samples were then separated by centrifugation and plasma frozen at -20°C until assayed for total bupivacaine. If possible (i.e. enough plasma), free bupivacaine concentrations were also measured.

Plasma bupivacaine (total and free) analysis

Total plasma bupivacaine concentrations were determined by addition of 100 ng of pentycaine to 200 µl of plasma followed by addition of 200 µl of 0.5 M NaOH. The sample was extracted with ethyl acetate, the solvent was removed and the residue was dissolved in 0.5 ml of 0.1 M phosphate buffer at pH 3.0. The sample was passed through a SCX (strong cation exchange) solid phase extraction cartridge (Isolute SCX, Crawford Scientific, Strathaven, Lanarkshire, UK) and was eluted with 1 M ammonia in methanol (1 ml). It was then blown to dryness and dissolved in ethyl acetate (0.1 ml) for analysis by gas chromatography-mass spectrometry (GC-MS). The GC-MS analysis was carried out using a Hewlett-Packard HP5988A GC-MS system in the electron impact (EI) mode; selected ion monitoring (SIM) was carried out for ions at m/z 140 for bupivacaine. The GC was fitted with a HP-1 column, helium was used as a carrier gas at a pressure of 40 kPa and the GC oven was programmed as follows: 100°C for 1 min and 20°C/min increments to 320°C.

For analysis of the free plasma bupivacaine concentration an aliquot of plasma (200 µl) was diluted with 20 µl of 1 M phosphate buffer and was centrifuged (1000 g) in a Centrifree MPS ultrafiltration unit (Millipore, Watford, UK). The ultrafiltrate was collected and 10 ng of pentycaine internal standard were added. The sample was then processed as described above (13, 14).

Pharmacokinetic analysis

For each infant, the maximal total plasma concentration (C_{MAX}) and time to maximal plasma concentration (T_{MAX}) were determined. The free plasma bupivacaine concentrations were measured in each individual sample over time in 3 infants from both groups. The free fraction (f_μ) was calculated from the free concentration and the total concentration from measurements of 3-6 samples from each individual; f_μ data from both groups were pooled to calculate an average value for all children.

In those infants in whom a consistent decline in plasma bupivacaine concentration with time was seen (Fig. 1) an "apparent" terminal half-life (t1/2) was calculated using the equation: EQUATION

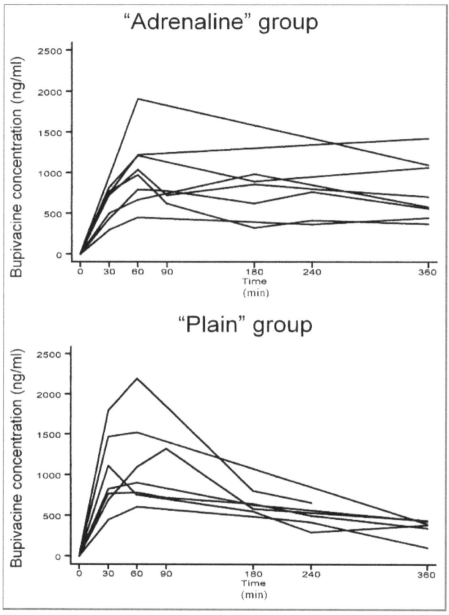

Fig. 1. The individual plasma bupivacaine concentration-time profiles from all the infants in both the "plain" group and the "adrenaline" group.

$$K_{el} = \frac{(\ln C_1 - \ln C_2)}{T_2 - T_1} = \frac{\Delta \ln C}{\Delta \ln T} = >t\frac{1}{2} = \frac{\ln 2}{K_{el}}$$

Equation 1

Statistical analysis

All data are stated as median (range). Between group comparison was made with Mann-Whitney's U-test. A P-value <0.05 was considered statistically significant.

Results

Fifteen ASA I or II children (all boys) were included in this study. Demographic details and surgical procedures are listed in Table 1. The duration of anaesthesia was comparable in both groups. In the "plain" group, the anaesthetic lasted a median of 35 min (range 25-70 min) as opposed to a median of 45 min (range 30-55 min) in the "adrenaline" group. Similarly, the duration of surgery also was comparable in both groups. In the "plain" group, surgery lasted a median of 25 min (range 15-55 min) as opposed to a median of 32.5 min (range 20-45 min) in the "adrenaline" group. Seven infants received plain bupivacaine and eight infants received bupivacaine with adrenaline (1/400 000). The caudal blocks were considered successful in all infants as they achieved adequate intra- and postoperative analgesia. No clinical signs of systemic toxicity were seen in any infant. None of the infants required any additional analgesia during the study period.

Demographic details, median (range).

Plain group					Adrenaline group				
Patient no.	Age (weeks)	PCA (weeks)	Weight (kg)	Surgery	Patient no.	Age (weeks)	PCA (weeks)	Weight (kg)	Surgery
1	5	45	4.9	RIH	1	22	62	7.0	RIH
2	10	38	2.5	LIH	2	10	44	3.4	RIH
3	14	54	7.1	Vesicostomy	3	16	56	6.9	BIH
4	22	61	7.3	RIH	4	12	51	6.3	RIH
5	14	52	5.1	RIH	5	14	47	4.3	BIH
6	14	46	4.4	RIH	6	5	45	4.0	RIH
7	10	48	4.7	RIH	7	0.6	40	3.0	BIH
					8	10	41	2.9	BIH
Median	14	48	4.9			11	46	4.15	
(range)	(5-22)	(38-61)	(2.5-7.3)			(0.6-22)	(40-62)	(2.9-7.0)	

Abbreviations: PCA=post conceptual age, LIH, RIH and BIH=left-, right- and bilateral herniotomy.

Table 1 Demographic details, median (range).

Overall, the total plasma bupivacaine concentrations in all but one sample were below 2 µg/ml. This sample was taken at t=60 min in a 14-week-old term baby and found to be 2195 ng/ml. The total bupivacaine levels ranged between 114 ng/ml and 2196 ng/ml. No differences in the total plasma bupivacaine concentrations could be found at any of the time points from 30 min to 240 min. However, the median total bupivacaine concentration at t=360 min was significantly higher in the "adrenaline" group compared to the "plain" group, i.e. 742 ng/ml (372-1423 ng/ml) vs. 400.5 ng/ml (114-446 ng/ml), $P=0.0080$. No differences in C_{MAX} or T_{MAX} could be found between the groups. The plasma concentration-time profiles for both groups are shown in Fig. 1. The measurements of free bupivacaine were made on individual samples in 3 infants from both groups. Due to small numbers no differences were found in the free bupivacaine concentrations between the groups. Overall, the free levels remained fairly stable throughout the study period, ranging between 13 ng/ml and 52 ng/ml. The corresponding median percentage of free bupivacaine (f_u) was 2.8% (1.3-4.6%) in the "plain" and 3.2% (1.3-6.7%) in the "adrenaline" group. When looking at both groups, the combined median f_u was 3.0% (1.3-6.7%).

The median "apparent" terminal half-life (t 1/2) was found to be significantly longer in the "adrenaline"

8   5/7/08 15:54

group (n=5), i.e. 363 min (range 238-537 min) compared to 165 min (range 104-264 min) in the plain group (n=6), P=0.0087.

The pharmacokinetic parameters are detailed in Table 2.

Pharmacokinetic parameters, median (range)			
		Plain group	Adrenaline group
	T_{MAX} (min)	60 (30–240)	60 (60–360)
	C_{MAX} (ng/ml)	1109 (607–2195)	1012 (449–1909)
	K_{e}* (min^{-1})	0.00420 (0.00240–0.00665)	0.00220 (0.00115–0.00291)
	$t_{\frac{1}{2}}$** (min)	165 (104–264) (n=6)	363 (238–537) (n=5)
	C_{360}*** (ng/ml)	400.5 (114–446)	742 (372–1423)
* P=0.00152			
** P=0.0087			
*** P=0.0080			

Table 2 Pharmacokinetic parameters, median (range).

Discussion

This is the first study describing the effects of adrenaline on the systemic absorption and pharmacokinetics of caudally administered bupivacaine in infants. Although the effects of adrenaline to a great extent depend on the site of the injection, it may also depend on the local anaesthetic agent, as well as the concentration used (15).

In theory, when using longer acting lipophilic local anaesthetic drugs such as bupivacaine, the effects of adrenaline tend to be less obvious than with hydrophilic drugs, such as lignocaine. It is believed that bupivacaine when injected epidurally will bind to the epidural fat and subsequently is released slowly. However, small babies have less epidural fat and a much higher cardiac output, and due to the relatively short-acting actions of adrenaline the systemic absorption lowering effects of adrenaline may be negligible (1, 15).

In this study, the total plasma bupivacaine concentrations measured were below 2 μg/ml in all but one sample, irrespective of the group. Surprisingly, the addition of adrenaline to the local anaesthetic solution did not influence the C_{MAX} obtained.

Interestingly, however, we were able to show a prolonged systemic absorption of bupivacaine in infants receiving a caudal block with 0.25% bupivacaine with 1:400 000 adrenaline compared to plain 0.25% bupivacaine. This was manifested by a significantly higher median total plasma bupivacaine concentration at t=360 min in the "adrenaline" group 742 ng/ml (range 372-1423 ng/ml) vs. 400.5 ng/ml (range 114-446 ng/ml) in the "plain" group. The resulting mean "apparent" terminal half-life, too, was significantly prolonged in the "adrenaline" group, i.e. 363 min (range 238-537 min) vs. 165 min (104-264 min) in the "plain" group.

The aim of this study was to investigate the effects of adrenaline on the systemic absorption of caudal bupivacaine and we did not attempt to estimate the clinical effects - if any.

In a study from 1988 by Mazoit et al., the pharmacokinetics of caudal bupivacaine was examined in 13 infants aged 1-6 months of age. They found peak plasma concentrations (C_{MAX}) of between 550 ng/ml and 1930 ng/ml after 10-60 min (T_{MAX}) and a mean terminal half-life (t 1/2) of 462 min (range 216-654 min). The mean free unbound bupivacaine concentration was 140 ng/ml (range 50-210 ng/ml) and the corresponding mean free fraction (f_u) was 0.16 (range 0.08-0.31) (5). In the present study the free bupivacaine concentrations were somewhat lower ranging between 13 ng/ml and 52 ng/ml, as were the corresponding f_u ranging between 1.3% and 6.7% (i.e. comparable to levels reported in adults). The reasons for this discrepancy may be many. First of all, the degree of binding varies significantly from individual to individual. Furthermore, intra-individually, the free levels may vary with the total levels. Since the [alpha]$_1$-acid glycoprotein levels continue to rise postoperatively (being an acute phase protein), the level of free drug might fall as the total level rises, depending on the relationship between the pharmacokinetics of the drug and the variation in $[alpha]_1$-acid glycoprotein levels. In addition, problems associated with the different methodologies used may be of importance too. Basically, there are three methods, which are applicable to the measurement of the free and the bound form of a drug: equilibrium dialysis, ultrafiltration and microdialysis. All of these methods suffer from drawbacks. The extent of protein binding is a function of drug and protein concentrations, the affinity constant for the drug-protein interaction, and the number of protein binding sites per class of binding site. Ultimately, as in all methods, the question remains as to how much the separation process perturbs the equilibrium between the free and bound forms of the drug (13, 16). It must be stressed, however, that there are not many measurements in neonates and infants to compare with in the literature. In a recent work by our group, utilising micro-equilibrium dialysis, we have found that the free levels of bupivacaine are in the range of 2-2.5% in neonates, despite $[alpha]_1$-acid glycoprotein levels being lower than in adults (Watson DG, personal communication). The problems of protein binding and bupivacaine in neonates/infants are an important issue that needs further attention.

In another study comprising older children (n=6) aged between 5.5 and 10 years of age, total C_{MAX} values between 960 ng/ml and 1640 ng/ml at T_{MAX} between 19.7 min and 38.4 min and a mean t 1/2 of 277 min (range 175-377 min) was reported (4).

The adrenaline concentration used in this study 1/400 000 (=2.5 µg/ml) was chosen for two reasons. Firstly, the desired concentration of both bupivacaine and adrenaline was easily prepared from the manufacturer's solution of 0.5% bupivacaine with 1/200 000 adrenaline by diluting this solution 1:1 with normal saline prior to the caudal injection. Secondly, during the preparation of the project claims had been made as to direct toxic effects to the medulla from high local adrenaline concentrations, resulting in ischaemic injuries to the medulla (1, 15).

The sample size in this study was fairly small (n=15 in total) as were the numbers of blood samples taken. The latter was a restriction from our local Ethics Committee, which only allowed us to take a total volume of blood of 1 ml/kg for research purposes from each child. Our results, however, are in keeping with those of other investigators - albeit the median t 1/2 in this study was somewhat shorter at 165 min and 363 min, respectively, compared to the findings by Mazoit et al. (mean t 1/2=462 min) (5). By looking at Fig. 1, it seems obvious that the addition of adrenaline to bupivacaine results in a prolonged absorption phase within the study period. What happens beyond 360 min remains to be elucidated.

C_{MAX} and T_{MAX} are highly context dependent parameters, hence these results should be interpreted with caution, but the results in this study are not much different to those reported by other investigators.

In conclusion, this study using pharmacokinetic parameters confirms that the addition of 1/400 000 adrenaline prolongs the systemic absorption of caudally administered bupivacaine in infants.

References

1. Rowney DA, Doyle E. Epidural and subarachnoid blockade in children. *Anaesthesia* 1998: **53**: 980-1001. [Context Link]

2. Dalens B, Hasnaoui A. Caudal anesthesia in pediatric surgery: success rate and adverse effects in 750 consecutive patients. *Anesth Analg* 1989: **68**: 83-89. [Context Link]

3. Arthur DS, McNicol LR. Local anaesthetic technique in paediatric surgery. *Br J Anaesth* 1986: **58**: 760-778. SFX| Bibliographic Links| [Context Link]

4. Ecoffey C, Desparmet J, Berdaux A, Maury M, Giudecelli SF, Saint-Maurice C. Bupivacaine in children - pharmacokinetics following caudal anesthesia. *Anesthesiology* 1988: **69**: 102-106. [Context Link]

　　　5/7/08 15:54

5. Mazoit JX, Denson DD, Saimii K. Pharmacokinetics of bupivacaine following caudal anesthesia in infants. *Anesthesiology* 1988: **68:** 387-391. SFX| Bibliographic Links| [Context Link]

6. Eyres RL, Bishop W, Oppenheim RC, Brown TCK. Plasma bupivacaine concentrations in children during caudal anaesthesia. *Anaesthesia Intensive Care* 1983: **11:** 20-22. SFX| Bibliographic Links| [Context Link]

7. Eyres RL, Kidd J, Oppenheim R, Brown TCK. Local anaesthetic plasma levels in children. *Anaesthesia Intensive Care* 1978: **6:** 243-247. SFX| Bibliographic Links| [Context Link]

8. Takasaki M. Blood concentrations of lidocaine, mepivacaine and bupivacaine during caudal analgesia in children. *Acta Anaesthesiol Scand* 1984: **28:** 211-214. SFX| Bibliographic Links| [Context Link]

9. Lerman J, Strong AS, LeDez KM, Swartz J, Rieder MJ, Burrows FA. Effects of age on the serum concentrations of [alpha]$_1$-acid glycoprotein and the binding of lidocaine in pediatric patients. *Clin Pharmacol Ther* 1989: **46:** 219-225. [Context Link]

10. Berde CB. Toxicity of local anesthetics in infants and children. *J Pediatr* 1993: **122:** S14-S20. SFX| Bibliographic Links| [Context Link]

11. Warner MA, Kunkel SE, Offord KO, Atchison SR, Dawson B. The effects of age, epinephrine and operative site on duration of caudal analgesia in pediatric patients. *Anesth Analg* 1987: **66:** 995-998. SFX| Ovid Full Text| Bibliographic Links| [Context Link]

12. Fischer QA, McComiskey CM, Hill JL et al. Postoperative voiding interval and duration of analgesia following peripheral or caudal block in children. *Anesth Analg* 1993: **76:** 173-177. [Context Link]

13. Stakim M, Watson DG, Morton NS, Hansen TG. Some difficulties in the separation of bound and unbound forms of bupivacaine in plasma using ultrafiltration. *J Pharm Pharmacol* 1997: **49:** A25. [Context Link]

14. Tahroui A, Watson DG, Skellern GG, Hudson SA, Petrie P. Comparative study of the determination of bupivacaine in human plasma by gas-chromatography mass spectrometry and high performance liquid chromatography. *J Pharm Biomed Anal* 1996: **15:** 251-257. SFX| Full Text| Bibliographic Links| [Context Link]

15. Cook B, Doyle E. The use of additives to local anaesthetic solutions for caudal epidural blockade. *Paediatr Anaesth* 1996: **6:** 353-359. SFX| Bibliographic Links| [Context Link]

16. Wright JD, Boudinot FD, Ujhelyi MR. Measurement and analysis of unbound drug concentrations. *Clin Pharmacokinet* 1996: **30:** 445-462. SFX| Bibliographic Links| [Context Link]

Key words: Local anesthetic: bupivacaine; anesthetic technique: caudal block; pharmacokinetics: systemic absorption, neonates and infants

---

Full Text

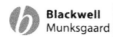

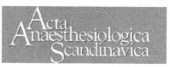

Plasma paracetamol concentrations and pharmacokinetics following rectal administration in neonates and young infants

Author(s):	Hansen, T. G.[1]; O'Brien, K.[1]; Morton, N. S.[1]; Rasmussen, S. N.[2]	ISSN: 0001-5172 Accession: 10492416
Issue:	Volume 43(8), September 1999, pp 855-859	
Publication Type:	[General Anaesthesia]	
Publisher:	© 1999 The Acta Anaesthesiologica Foundation.	
Institution(s):	[1]Directorate of Anaesthesia, The Royal Hospital for Sick Children, Glasgow, Scotland, United Kingdom and [2]Department of Biological Sciences, The Royal Danish School of Pharmacy, Copenhagen, Denmark Received 17 August 1998, accepted for publication 3 May 1999 Address: Dr Neil S. Morton; Dept. of Anaesthesia; Royal Hospital for Sick Children, Yorkhill; Glasgow G3 8SJ, Scotland; United Kingdom	

Keywords: Absorption, Acetaminophen, Acetaminophen, Acetaminophen, Administration, Rectal, Analgesics, Non-Narcotic, Analgesics, Non-Narcotic, Analgesics, Non-Narcotic, Anesthesia, General, Anesthesia, Local, Body Weight, Colorimetry, Female, Follow-Up Studies, Half-Life, Humans, Infant, Infant, Newborn, Male, Suppositories

Abstract

Background: Despite widespread use in children pharmacokinetic data about paracetamol are relatively scarce, not the least in the youngest age groups. This study aimed to describe plasma paracetamol concentrations and pharmacokinetics of a single rectal paracetamol dose in neonates and young infants.

Methods: Perioperatively, 17 neonates and infants <=160 days of age received one rectal paracetamol dose (mean 23.9 mg/kg (±4.2 mg/kg)). Blood samples were drawn at 60, 120, 180, 240, 300 and 360 min, according to the infants' weights. Plasma paracetamol concentrations were measured by a Colorometric Assay, Ectachem Clinical Chemistry Slides (Johnson & Johnson Clinical Diagnostics).

Results: The plasma paracetamol concentrations were mainly below the therapeutic (i.e. antipyretic) range of 66-132 µmol/l and did not exceed 160 µmol/l in any infant. The mean maximum plasma concentration (C_{max}) was 72.4 µmol/l (±33.5 µmol/l) and the time to C_{max}, i.e. the mean T_{max} was 102.4 min (±59.1 min). The mean "apparent" terminal half-life (n=10) was 243.6 min (±114.1 min).

Conclusion: The absorption of rectal paracetamol (mean dose 23.9 mg/kg, ±4.2mg/kg) in young infants <160 days is variable and often prolonged and achieves mainly subtherapeutic plasma concentrations.

Paracetamol is the most widely used analgesic and antipyretic in children. It is a drug with few contraindications and few adverse effects when used in recommended doses. In addition, it can be administered by the oral, rectal and intravenous routes (1-4). Paracetamol acts by inhibiting peripheral and central prostaglandin synthesis but, unlike the non-steroidal anti-inflammatory drugs (NSAIDS), it has weak anti-inflammatory properties (5). A "ceiling effect" is seen for analgesia with paracetamol (6).

The plasma paracetamol concentration range associated with an anti-pyretic effect is 66-132 µl/l (10-20 mg/l; conversion factor is 6.6 µmol/mg) (1,2). The optimal analgesic plasma concentration range may be somewhat higher, but has not been clearly defined (7).

Hepatotoxicity occurs when peak plasma concentration is approximately 10-times this level, at around 990 µmol/l (8). The minimum potentially toxic single dose in children has been calculated as 150 mg/kg (9), but may be less in those with renal disease, hepatic disease, dehydration or malnutrition.

When administered orally, paracetamol is well absorbed within 30-60 min and therapeutic plasma concentrations are maintained for 2-4 h after a single dose of 15-20 mg/kg (10). After rectal administration, the relative bioavailability is poor and absorption is slow and erratic with an average time to reach maximum plasma concentration (T_{max}) of 2.3 h (3,8,11-14). It has been demonstrated that a rectal loading dose of 40-45 mg/kg is needed to achieve and sustain therapeutic plasma concentrations in children older than 1 year (7,14,15). However, pharmacokinetic data are sparse in the youngest age groups (4,13,16-18), and our study aimed to describe the plasma concentration time profile and pharmacokinetics of a single rectal dose of paracetamol in neonates and young infants.

Methods

Following ethical approval and written informed parental consent, neonates and infants less than 160 days of age scheduled for minor surgery were enrolled in the study. Infants who had received paracetamol within the previous 24 h were excluded, as were infants with any known renal or hepatic impairments. After induction, but before the start of surgery, all infants received a single rectal paracetamol dose of approximately 25 mg/kg. The paracetamol (Alvedon®, Novex Pharma Ltd., Marlow, UK) given was formulated in a stearate-based suppository and used in a strength of either 60 mg or 125 mg.

Anaesthetic technique

Apart from EMLA, no premedication was given and all infants received a standardized non-opioid-based general anaesthetic technique, supplemented with an appropriate regional block.

The general anaesthetic technique comprised induction with thiopenthone (3-5 mg/kg) and suxamethonium (1.0-1.5 mg/kg) or atracurium (0.5 mg/kg). Following endotracheal intubation, the infants' lungs, were ventilated to normocapnia with 50% oxygen in nitrous oxide and desflurane. Eleven infants received a caudal block with bupivacaine 0.25% (1.0 ml/kg), 4 infants received wound infiltration with bupivacaine 0.25% (0.25-0.5 ml/kg) and 1 infant received local anaesthetic eye drops with amethocaine 0.5%. One infant did not receive any local anaesthesia. No infants required any further analgesics during the study period.

After surgery, residual neuromuscular blockade was reversed with glycopyrrolate (10 µg/kg) and neostigmine

(50 µg/kg) and all children were extubated.

Blood sampling
Immediately after the anaesthetic induction, a dedicated peripheral intravenous cannula (venflon 22 G, Ohmeda, Sweden) was inserted in a saphenous vein for blood sampling. Patency of this cannula was maintained by an infusion of 5% glucose with 0.225% saline 3-5 ml/h.

Blood samples (0.7-1.0 ml/sample) were collected from the i.v. cannula at 60, 120, 180, 240, 300 and 360 min after the administration of the suppository. The total number of blood samples from each individual was restricted by the Ethics Committee's limit of 1 ml/kg, but it was possible to sample all infants at 60, 120 and 360 min. Older infants had additional samples drawn at intermediate time points according to weight. Blood samples were separated by centrifugation and the plasma was stored at -20°C until assay.

Paracetamol analysis
Plasma paracetamol levels were measured by a commercially available Colorometric Assay, the Ectachem Clinical Chemistry Slides (ACET) (Johnson & Johnson Clinical Diagnostics, Inc., New York, USA) according to the manufacturer's instruction. The accuracy of this method has been shown over a wide range of concentrations when compared with both a high-performance liquid chromatography (HPLC) and a fluorescence polarization reference technique. The sensitivity-limit of the assay was 25 µmol/l and the intraassay and interassay coefficient of variation of the method was <5%. No drugs known to interfere with the assay were given to any infants.

Pharmacokinetics
For each infant, we determined maximal plasma concentration (C_{max}) and time to maximal plasma concentration (T_{max}). Due to erratic or delayed absorption, the limited number of samples taken and the short duration of sampling time, we were unable to calculate detailed pharmacokinetic parameters in this study. However, in 10 infants in whom a consistent decline in plasma paracetamol with time was seen (Fig. 1), we calculated an "apparent" terminal half-life (t½), using the equation: $k_e = (\ln C_1 - \ln C_2)/T_2 - T_1 = [DELTA]\ln C/[DELTA]T$ [right double arrow] $t½ = \ln 2/k_e$, from two or more data points between 60 and 360 min, assuming a terminated absorption phase.

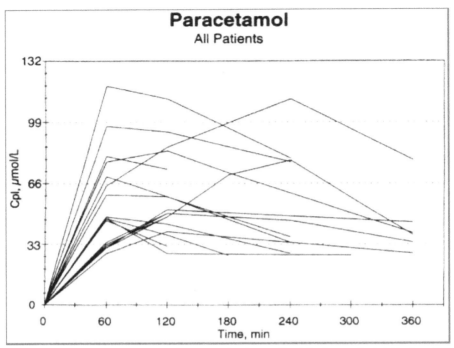

Fig. 1. The individual plasma paracetamol concentration-time profiles following rectal administration of 23.9 mg/kg (±4.1 mg/kg) paracetamol in neonates and infants, omitting plasma levels <25 μmol/l.

The C_{max} obtained was correlated to the actual paracetamol dose given (range 17.6-32.8 mg/kg) using linear regression.

Data are stated as mean (±SD). A P-value <0.05 was considered statistically significant.

Results

Seventeen neonates and young infants <=160 days of age were enrolled in this study (3 girls and 14 boys). Their mean postnatal ages were 71.5 days (±47 days) and their corresponding mean weights were 3.9 kg (±1.4 kg). Eight children had been born prematurely. Their mean gestational ages at birth were 32.6 weeks (±2.6 weeks) and at the time of the study their mean postconceptual ages were 39.8 weeks (±3.7 weeks). Demographic details and surgical procedures are listed in Table 1.

Patient	Sex M/F	Age days	T/P	Weight kg	Diagnosis	Operation
1	F	157	T	6.7	glaucoma	trabeculectomy
2	M	58	P	2.0	bilateral hernias	herniotomies
3	M	67	P	2.3	bilateral hernias	herniotomies
4	M	46	T	3.2	CPS	pylorotomy
5	M	73	P	3.4	RIH	herniotomy
6	M	26	P	2.8	CPS	pylorotomy
7	M	142	T	6.1	RIH	herniotomy
8	M	60	P	4.8	RIH	herniotomy
9	F	38	T	3.9	CPS	pylorotomy
10	M	160	T	5.8	CDH	reduction of CDH
11	M	124	P	3.6	bilateral hernias	herniotomies
12	M	2	T	2.6	SBA	ileostomy
13	M	60	P	2.5	lateral hernias	herniotomies
14	M	45	T	4.2	CPS	pylorotomy
15	F	44	T	5.0	imperforated hymen	opening
16	M	30	P	3.0	bilateral hernias	herniotomies
17	M	84	T	5.0	RIH	herniotomy

Abbreviations. M = male, F = female, T = baby born at term, P = baby born prematurely, SBA = small bowel atresia, CDH = congenital dysplasia of hip, CPS = congenital pyloric stenosis, RIH = right inguinal hernia.

Table 1 Demographic data.

The mean paracetamol dose administered to the infants in this study was 23.9 mg/kg (±4.2 mg/kg). The resulting plasma paracetamol concentration/time profile for each individual is shown in Fig. 1. The plasma concentrations were mainly below the therapeutic "antipyretic" range and did not exceed 160 μmol/l in any infant (Fig. 1). The mean C_{max} was 72.4 μmol/l (±33.5 μmol/l) and the corresponding time to obtain C_{max}, i.e. the mean T_{max}, was 102.4 min (±59.1 min). In those 10 infants in whom we were able to calculate an "apparent" terminal half-life (t½), we found a mean t½ of 243.6 min (±114.1 min).

The relationship between C_{max} and the actual paracetamol dose given is shown in Fig. 2 (C_{max}=2.71×Dose+1.52; r^2=0.264, P<0.05).

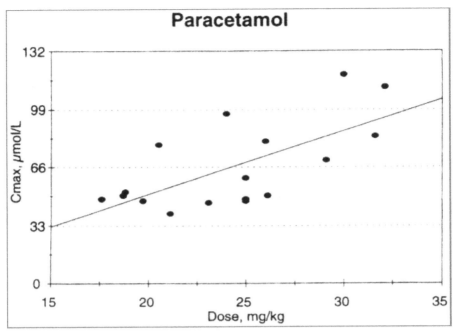

Fig. 2. The relationship between the actual paracetamol dose given (range 17.6-32.8 mg/kg) and the C_{max} obtained (C_{max}=2.71×Dose+1.52; r^2=0.264, P<0.05).

Discussion

This study showed an incomplete or delayed absorption of 23.9 mg/kg (±4.2 mg/kg) rectal paracetamol in young infants <=160 days of age. The resulting mean plasma concentrations were subtherapeutic (i.e. less than 66-132 µmol/l). The mean C_{max} was 72.4 µmol/l (±33.5 µmol/l) and the corresponding time to obtain C_{max}, i.e. the mean T_{max} was 102.4 min (±59.1 min). The accuracy of the pharmacokinetic data obtained in this study may be somewhat unreliable due to the limited number of blood samples in many of the children. However, the results are in keeping with those of other investigators, though comprising mainly older children (4,7,11-16). Following rectal paracetamol doses of 18.1 mg/kg (13) and 20 mg/kg (16), mean C_{max} levels of 52.1 µmol/l and 55.4 µmol/l at T_{max} of 58 min and 78 min have been demonstrated in 2 studies comprising 9 and 5 neonates, respectively. In another study comprising 10 infants receiving a mean rectal paracetamol dose of 17.9 mg/kg, a mean C_{max} of 37.6 µmol/l at a T_{max} of 78 min was obtained (13).

We were able to estimate an "apparent" mean terminal half-life of 243.6 min (±114.1 min) in 10 of the infants studied. We must emphasize that the assumption held for the t½ calculated in this study, i.e. a completed absorption phase before T_1 and T_2, may not necessarily be fulfilled. However, application of the Wagner-Nelson method (19) to the profiles from 8 of these 10 patients gives a mean absorption half-life of 18.7 min (±9.9 min). This indicates that when the elimination constant is calculated from data points from 120 min and onwards, 99% of the absorption has already occurred. Furthermore, our results are comparable to previous studies comprising neonates and young infants reporting mean elimination half-lives of 168-294 min (4,13,17,18). Interestingly, in infancy shorter elimination half-lives have been reported (96-126 min) (13,17).

Several factors may contribute to the incomplete or delayed absorption of rectal paracetamol. The relative bioavailability of a suppository may furthermore depend on the formulation, i.e. the absorption of lipophilic suppositories are more rapid than that of hydrophilic suppositories (21). The height in the rectum may be important in small children. The suppository is relatively large in relation to the rectum of the smaller infant. This could mean that a major part is absorbed via the superior rectal venous drainage directly into the portal vein and thus undergo a significant first-pass hepatic clearance. Other factors known to interfere with rectal absorption of drugs are: pH, defaecation, the contents of the rectal vaults and the colonic blood flow. The anaesthetics (mainly the inhalational agents) may reduce the colonic blood flow and thereby delay absorption (3,4,7,12,15).

Furthermore, the rate at which suppositories dissolve may be a function of suppository dose size, in that smaller dose suppositories dissolve more rapidly (11). Interestingly, high rectal paracetamol doses are not accompanied by a shorter T_{max} (7,11,14,15).

In conclusion, the absorption of 23.9 mg/kg (±4.2 mg/kg) of rectally administered paracetamol is variable and often prolonged in young infants <=160 days of age. The resulting plasma concentrations are mainly subtherapeutic and the mean "apparent" terminal t½ is 243.6 min (±114.1 min).

References

1. Walson PD, Mortensen ME. Pharmacokinetics of common analgesics, anti-inflammatories and antipyretics in children. *Clin Pharmacokinet* 1989: **17** (suppl. 1): 116-137. [Context Link]

2. Wilson JT, Brown RD, Bocchini Jr JA, Kerans GL. Efficacy, disposition and pharmacodynamics of aspirin, acetaminophen and choline salicylate in young febrile children. *Ther Drug Monit* 1982: **4**: 147-180. SFX| Bibliographic Links | [Context Link]

3. Seideman P, Alvan G, Andrews RS, Labross A. Relative bio-availability of a paracetamol suppository. *Eur J Clin Pharmacol* 1980: **17**: 465-468. [Context Link]

4. Miller RP, Roberts RJ, Fischer LJ. Acetaminophen elimination kinetics in neonates, children and adults. *Clin Pharmacol Ther* 1976: **19**: 284-294. SFX| Bibliographic Links | [Context Link]

5. Piletta P, Porchet HC, Dayer P. Distinct central nervous system involvement of paracetamol and salicylate. In: Bond MR, Charlton JE, Woolf CJ (eds). Proceedings of the 6th World Congress on Pain. Adelaide: Elsevier Science Publishers BV, 1991: 181-184. [Context Link]

6. Anderson B, Kanagasundarum K, Woolard G. Analgesic efficacy of paracetamol in children using tonsillectomy as a pain model. *Anaesth Intensive Care* 1997: **24**: 669-673. [Context Link]

7. Anderson BJ, Woolard GA, Holford NHG. Pharmacokinetics of rectal paracetamol after major surgery in children. *Paediatr Anaesth* 1995: **5**: 237-242. SFX| Bibliographic Links | [Context Link]

8. Prescott LF, Roscoe P, Wright N et al. Plasma paracetamol half-life in patients with paracetamol overdosage. *Lancet* 1971: **I**: 519-522. [Context Link]

9. Jackson CH, MacDonald NC, Cornett JWD. Acetaminophen: a practical pharmacologic overview. *Can Med Assoc J* 1984: **131**: 25-37. SFX| Full Text| Bibliographic Links | [Context Link]

10. Adithan C, Thangham J. A comparative study of saliva and serum paracetamol using a simple spectrophotometric study. *Br J Clin Pharmacol* 1982: **14**: 107-109. SFX| Bibliographic Links | [Context Link]

11. Birmingham PK, Tobin MJ, Henthorn TK et al. Twenty-four hour pharmacokinetics of rectal acetaminophen in children: an old drug with new recommendations. *Anesthesiology* 1997: **87**: 244-252. SFX| Ovid Full Text| Bibliographic Links | [Context Link]

12. Gaudreault P, Guay J, Nicol O, Dupuis G. Pharmacokinetics and clinical efficacy of intrarectal solution of acetaminophen. *Can J Anaesth* 1988: **35**: 149-152. SFX| Bibliographic Links| [Context Link]

13. Hopkins CS, Underhill S, Booker PD. Pharmacokinetics of paracetamol after cardiac surgery. *Arch Dis Child* 1990: **65**: 971-976. SFX| Bibliographic Links| [Context Link]

14. Houck CS, Sullivan LJ, Wilder RT et al. Pharmacokinetics of a higher dose of rectal acetaminophen in children. *Anesthesiology* 1996: **85**: A1126. [Context Link]

15. Montgomery CJ, McGormack JP, Reichert CC, Marsland CP. Plasma concentrations after high-dose (45 mg/kg) rectal acetaminophen in children. *Can J Anaesth* 1995: **45**: 982-986. [Context Link]

16. Lin Y-C, Sussman HH, Benitz WE. Plasma concentrations after rectal administration of acetaminophen in preterm neonates. *Paediatr Anaesth* 1997: **7**: 457-459. SFX| Bibliographic Links| [Context Link]

17. Autret E, Duherte JP, Bretau M et al. Pharmacokinetics of paracetamol in neonates after administration of propacetamol chlorhydrate. *Dev Pharmacol Ther* 1993: **20**: 129-134. SFX| Bibliographic Links| [Context Link]

18. Levy G, Khanna NN, Soda DM, Tsuzuki O, Stern L. Pharmacokinetics of acetaminophen in the human neonate: formation of acetaminophen glucuronide and sulphate in relation to plasma bilirubin concentration and d-glucaric excretion. *Pediatrics* 1975: **55**: 818-825. SFX| Full Text| Bibliographic Links |[Context Link]

19. Wagner JG. Fundamentals of clinical pharmacokinetics. Hamilton, Illinois, USA: Drug Intelligence Publications, Inc., 1975: 174. [Context Link]

20. Peterson RG, Rumack BH. Pharmacokinetics of acetaminophen in children. *Pediatrics* 1978: **62** (Part 2): 877-879. SFX| Full Text| Bibliographic Links |

21. Keinänen S, Hietula M, Similä S, Kouvalainen K. Antipyretic therapy. Comparison of rectal and oral paracetamol. *Eur J Clin Pharmacol* 1977: **12**: 77-80. SFX| Bibliographic Links| [Context Link]

22. Nahata, MC, Powell DA, Durrell DE, Miller MA. Acetaminophen accumulation in pediatric patients after repeated therapeutic doses. *Eur J Clin Pharmacol* 1984: **27**: 57-59. SFX| Bibliographic Links|

23. Granry JC, Rod B, Boccard E, Hermann P, Gendron A, Saint-Maurice C. Pharmacokinetics and antipyretic effects of an injectable pro-drug of paracetamol (propacetamol) in children. *Paediatr Anaesth* 1992: **2**: 291-295.

Key words: Analgesics: paracetamol; pharmacokinetics: rectal absorption, neonates and infants

---

Pediatric Anesthesia 2004 **14**: 856–860

Remifentanil vs fentanyl/morphine for pain and stress control during pediatric cardiac surgery

G. BELL MBChB FRCA*, U. DICKSON MBChB FRCA†, A. ARANA
MBChB FRCA‡, D. ROBINSON MBChB FRCA*, C. MARSHALL
FRCA§ AND N. MORTON, MBChB FRCA FRCPCH*

*Department of Anaesthetics, The Royal Hospital for Sick Children, Yorkhill, Glasgow, UK,
†Department of Anaesthetics, Children's Hospital, Steelhouse Lane, Birmingham, UK,
‡Department of Anaesthetics, Leeds General Infirmary, Great George Street, Leeds, UK and
§Department of Anaesthetics, Middlemore Hospital Private Bag, Otahuhu, Auckland, New
Zealand*

Summary

Background: Remifentanil is a short acting, potent synthetic opioid that
does not accumulate after infusion or repeated bolus doses. It may be
rapidly titrated to the requirements of individual patients. Titrated
infusion of remifentanil may be able to provide potent analgesia
required for pediatric cardiac surgery and obtund the stress response
in theater whilst not having the persistent respiratory depression and
sedation seen with longer acting opioids.
Methods: Twenty patients were randomized to receive a titrated
infusion of remifentanil ($0–1$ $\mu g \cdot kg^{-1} \cdot min^{-1}$) or a standard dose of
fentanyl (30 $\mu g \cdot kg^{-1}$) prebypass plus morphine (1 $mg \cdot kg^{-1}$) on rewarming. Blood samples for glucose and cortisol were taken at regular
intervals from induction through bypass and into the first 24 h of
postoperative intensive care. In addition to biochemical indicators of
the stress response we recorded baseline hemodynamic parameters
and any acute physiological events.
Results: Ten patients received morphine, seven received remifentanil.
There were no statistically significant differences between the two
treatment groups in cortisol measurements, mean arterial pressure or
heart rate recordings. In the last time period the remifentanil group
had a larger rise in blood glucose concentration (baseline 3.9, rise
3 $mmol \cdot l^{-1}$) than the fentanyl/morphine group (baseline 4.2 rise
1.9 $mmol \cdot l^{-1}$), CI -4.3 to -0.2.
Conclusions: The only significant difference was in glucose in the
postbypass time periods. Although statistically significant, this difference is insufficient evidence of increased stress in the remifentanil
group. The results show that in the patients studied there was no
clinically important difference between the two techniques.

Keywords: congenital heart disease; remifentanil; stress response

Correspondence to: Dr G. Bell MBChB FRCA, Department of Anaesthetics, The Royal Hospital for Sick Children, Yorkhill, Glasgow, G3 8SJ, UK.
(email: graham.bell@yorkhill.scot.nhs.uk).

Introduction

Remifentanil is a selective μ-opioid receptor agonist. A synthetic piperidine derivative, it is around 16 times more potent than alfentanil (1). Nonspecific tissue and plasma esterases hydrolyze remifentanil into metabolites that are excreted by the kidney and have no significant clinical actions. The biological half-life of remifentanil is between 3 and 10 min; it has a fast onset of action and does not accumulate after infusion or repeated bolus administration (2), (3). These characteristics combine to give a theoretical clinical advantage of a potent opioid that can be rapidly titrated to meet the immediate clinical requirement and obtund the stress response to surgical stimulus, without persistent effects that may delay postoperative progress.

Methods

After approval by the local ethics committee, 20 patients who were scheduled for open-heart surgery were randomized to one of two treatment groups. Apart from the choice of opioid analgesia used, the anesthetic technique was that normally used by the consultant anesthetist in charge of the case. All patients had 5% glucose with saline 0.45% commenced before rewarming from cardiopulmonary bypass. Patients were excluded if they received steroids, or glucose infusions before cardiopulmonary bypass. The fentanyl and morphine group had a standard dose of fentanyl (30 $\mu g \cdot kg^{-1}$) incrementally prior to institution of cardiopulmonary bypass. This group also received morphine (1 $mg \cdot kg^{-1}$) on rewarming and had a morphine infusion commenced on admission to the intensive care unit. The remifentanil group received a remifentanil infusion (at a rate of 0–1 $\mu g \cdot kg \cdot min^{-1}$ and additional boluses of 1 $\mu g \cdot kg^{-1}$ if required), titrated to the patients' clinical requirement as judged by the anesthetist present. This infusion was given through an additional peripheral intravenous line inserted solely for that purpose. It was intended to continue the remifentanil infusion for 24 h on the intensive care unit, but the infusion could be exchanged for morphine at the discretion of intensive care staff. The remifentanil was continued post bypass as it was proposed that there may be advantages in titrating opioid requirements in the postbypass period and not because there was any attempt or desire to extubate the patient earlier in the postoperative period than those patients receiving fentanyl/morphine.

Heart rate and mean arterial pressure were recorded and averaged over time. In addition to these physiological variables, acute events such as tachycardia, bradycardia, or any changes that may have related to excessive or inadequate analgesia were recorded. Blood samples for glucose and cortisol were taken at regular intervals from before induction of anesthesia into the period of postoperative intensive care. Immediately after collection the specimens for cortisol were centrifuged and the serum was withdrawn for analysis.

For analysis purposes data were divided into three time periods: prebypass; during bypass and postbypass until admission to the intensive care unit.

For each biochemical or physiological parameter, the first recorded value was chosen as the baseline. This was a preinduction recording or sample in almost all cases. When it was not possible to withdraw blood from the peripheral cannula inserted with the child awake, a sample taken immediately postinduction was used as the baseline. The change from the baseline value to the maximum recorded value during each of the three time periods, was calculated. These changes were compared between the two groups using Mann–Whitney tests ($\alpha = 0.05$, unadjusted for multiple comparisons). All analyses were carried out using the statistical analysis package MINITAB Version 12.

Results

There were two late cancellations in the remifentanil group and one patient was also withdrawn from this group because of a protocol violation. One patient in the remifentanil group developed a junctional ectopic tachycardia following repair of an atrioventricular septal defect. Postoperative heart rate recordings were excluded from analysis for this patient. The details of cases presenting for surgical repair and the anesthetic techniques used are listed in Table 1.

Postbypass, patients in the remifentanil group had significantly higher glucose levels than those who received fentanyl/morphine [median difference from baseline −2.2, CI (−4.3, −0.2)] as shown in

© 2004 Blackwell Publishing Ltd, *Pediatric Anesthesia*, **14**, 856–860

Table 1
Details of cases presenting for repair and anesthetic technique

Operation	Age (months)	Preoperative condition/diagnoses	Anesthetic technique
Fentanyl and morphine group $n = 10$			
Tetralogy of Fallot repair	17	Desaturation on exertion supravalvular stenosis	Ketamine/rocuronium/isoflurane
Secundum atrial septal defect closure	48	Asymptomatic	Propofol/rocuronium/isoflurane
Sub aortic myectomy	28	Outflow tract gradient 80 mmHg	Sevoflurane/pancuronium/isoflurane
Tetralogy of Fallot repair	18	Good LV function, moderate right ventricular outflow tract obstruction	Ketamine/Vecuronium/Isoflurane
Atrial septectomy	39	Double outlet right ventricle, Glenn shunt planned but pulmonary pressure too high	Thiopentone/vecuronium/isoflurane
Ventricular septal defect closure	7	Presented with lethargy, pulmonary hypertension	Thiopentone/pancuronium/isoflurane
Ventricular septal defect closure	12	Presented with lethargy and failure to thrive, previous pulmonary artery band and coarctation repair	Sevoflurane/vecuronium/isoflurane
Ventricular septal defect closure	5	Presented with lethargy, pulmonary hypertension	Thiopentone/vecuronium/isoflurane
Atrioventricular septal defect repair	4	Downs syndrome, pulmonary hypertension	Sevoflurane/vecuronium/isoflurane
Secundum atrial septal defect closure	44	Moderate tricuspid regurgitation and partial anomalous pulmonary venous drainage	Propofol/pancuronium/isoflurane
Remifentanil group $n = 7$			
Secundum atrial septal defect closure	48	Low saturation, left superior vena cava	Propofol/pancuronium/isoflurane
Secundum atrial septal defect closure	35	Right ventricular enlargement	Thiopentone/pancuronium/isoflurane
Secundum atrial septal defect closure	35	Asymptomatic	Thiopentone/vecuronium/isoflurane
Secundum atrial septal defect closure	48	Mitral regurgitation & pulmonary stenosis	Thiopentone/vecuronium/isoflurane
Glenn shunt	53	Double outlet right ventricle, cyanosed, hypoplastic left ventricle, previous pulmonary artery band	Ketamine/vecuronium/isoflurane
Atrioventricular septal defect repair	3	Downs syndrome, in cardiac failure	Thiopentone/pancuronium/isoflurane
Secundum atrial septal defect closure	108	Downs syndrome, right ventricular enlargement	Thiopentone/vecuronium/isoflurane

Figure 1. There were no statistically significant differences between the two groups for other variables in any time period as illustrated in Figures 2, 3 and 4.

Two acute events occurred in the remifentanil group. One patient moved as cardiopulmonary bypass was commenced, requiring a bolus of remifentanil. This patient had received a single dose of vecuronium at induction, which had obviously worn off. Another patient became unsettled during transfer to intensive care. This was because of a kink in the peripheral cannula being used for the remifentanil infusion. Both of these events were accompanied by physiological change but neither caused identifiable changes in the biochemical measures of the stress response.

Four patients continued remifentanil infusions for 24 h in intensive care, the remaining three were converted to infusions of morphine during this period.

All patients were alive at routine follow up 1 year postoperatively.

Discussion and Conclusions

We conclude that the two techniques using either fentanyl/morphine or remifentanil produced broadly similar perioperative control of the stress response during open-heart surgery in children. Change from baseline measurement of heart rate, mean arterial pressure and serum cortisol were similar in both groups. Glucose levels were also similar before and during bypass, but were raised following bypass in the remifentanil group. Although statistically significant, we do not feel this change in glucose is clinically important. Taken

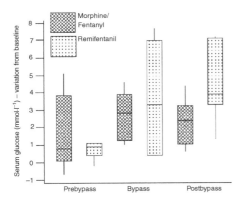

Figure 1
Box and whisker plot of change in serum glucose vs perioperative time period. Boxes represent interquartile range and whiskers represent maximal points that are not outliers.

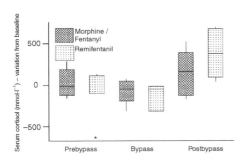

Figure 2
Box and whisker plot of change in serum cortisol vs perioperative time period. Boxes represent interquartile range and whiskers represent maximal points that are not outliers. Asterisks represent points that are >1.5 times the interquartile range.

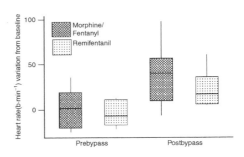

Figure 3
Box and whisker plot of change heart rate vs perioperative time period. Boxes represent interquartile range and whiskers represent maximal points that are not outliers.

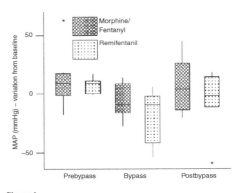

Figure 4
Box and whisker plot of change in mean arterial pressure vs perioperative time period. Boxes represent interquartile range and whiskers represent maximal points that are not outliers. Asterisks represent points that are >1.5 times the interquartile range.

alone a small rise in glucose is insufficient to indicate that the remifentanil patients were significantly more stressed than those in the fentanyl/morphine group.

It was intended to continue infusion of remifentanil for the first 24 h of intensive care. However, the majority of patients were converted to morphine infusions because of difficulty in achieving satisfactory sedation and analgesia, whilst also reestablishing spontaneous breathing. We would not recommend remifentanil infusion for sedation in the intensive care unit. The clearance of remifentanil is moderately increased in the postbypass period (4) this may contribute to the difficulty in selecting the required dose. There is interest in using remifentanil to facilitate early postoperative extubation but our study was not designed to assess the feasibility or timing of extubation.

The patient who moved when cardiopulmonary bypass was started highlights the large interindividual variation in dosage requirements. This patient was receiving the maximum rate of infusion used in our study and supplemental isoflurane. Although this dose has been found to be the ED50 for noncardiac surgery (5) using N_2O, O_2 and remifentanil technique, a rate of $1 \ \mu g \cdot kg^{-1} \cdot min^{-1}$ is not sufficient for all patients when the dilutional effects of cardiopulmonary bypass are imposed. Studies using remifentanil in combination with isoflurane for noncardiac surgery have found the average infusion rate required was $0.25 \ \mu g \cdot kg^{-1} \cdot min^{-1}$ (6).

Another practical problem was illustrated by the patient who moved when the infusion line was kinked. We would recommend that remifentanil infusions be given through a central line, when available to reduce the possibility of this happening. None of our study patients had bradycardia or hypotension although we commenced the remifentanil at a rate of $1 \ \mu g \cdot kg \cdot min^{-1}$ in most cases. This contrasts with findings in infants undergoing abdominal surgery (7).

Although we did not perform statistical analysis on the data once the patients had been admitted to the intensive care unit as the differences in treatment would have made the groups incomparable, patients from both groups showed similar patterns with serum cortisol measurements peaking around 18 h after admission to the intensive care unit. It may well be the case that both techniques simply delay the stress response as has been shown previously with other high dose opioid techniques.

Acknowledgements

Robertson Department of Statistics at Glasgow University. All consultant cardiac anesthetists and the Department of Biochemistry at the Royal Hospital for Sick Children, Yorkhill.

References

1 Egan TD, Minto C, Lemmens HJM et al. Remifentanil versus alfentanil: comparative pharmacodynamics. *Anesthesiology* 1994; **81:** A374.
2 Westmoreland CL, Hoke JF, Sebel P et al. Pharmacokinetics of remifentanil (GI87084B) and its major metabolite (GI920291) in patients undergoing elective inpatient surgery. *Anesthesiology* 1993; **79:** 893–903.
3 Glass PS, Hardman D, Kamiyama Y et al. Preliminary pharmacokinetics and pharmacodynamics of an ultra-short-acting opioid: remifentanil (G187084B). *Anesth Analg* 1993; **77:** 1031–1040.
4 Davis PJ, Wilson AS, Scierka MS et al. The effects of cardiopulmonary bypass on remifentanil kinetics in children undergoing atrial septal defect repair. *Anesth Analg* 1999; **89:** 904–908.
5 Davis PJ, Lerman J, Suresh S et al. A randomized multicentre study of remifentanil compared with alfentanil, isoflurane, or propofol in anesthetized pediatric patients undergoing elective strabismus surgery. *Anesth Analg* 1997; **84:** 982–989.
6 Prys-Roberts C, Lerman J, Murat I et al. Comparison of remifentanil versus regional anaesthesia in children anaesthetised with isoflrane/nitrous oxide. *Anaesthesia* 2000; **55:** 870–876.
7 Wee LH, Moriarty A, Cranston A et al. Remifentanil infusion for major abdominal surgery in infants. *Paediatr Anaesth* 1999; **9:** 415–418.

Accepted 12 December 2003

CPSIA information can be obtained
at www.ICGtesting.com
Printed in the USA
LVHW080549280223
740519LV00015B/263